KICK
THE FAT

A THREE-PART KICK-BOXING WORKOUT TO HELP YOU BURN FAT – FAST!

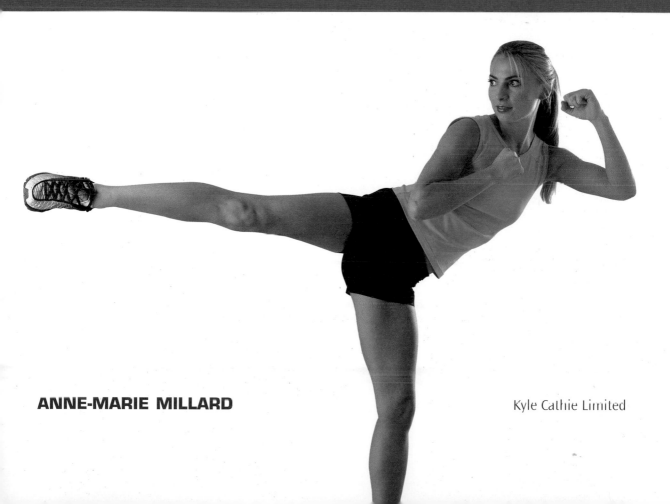

ANNE-MARIE MILLARD

Kyle Cathie Limited

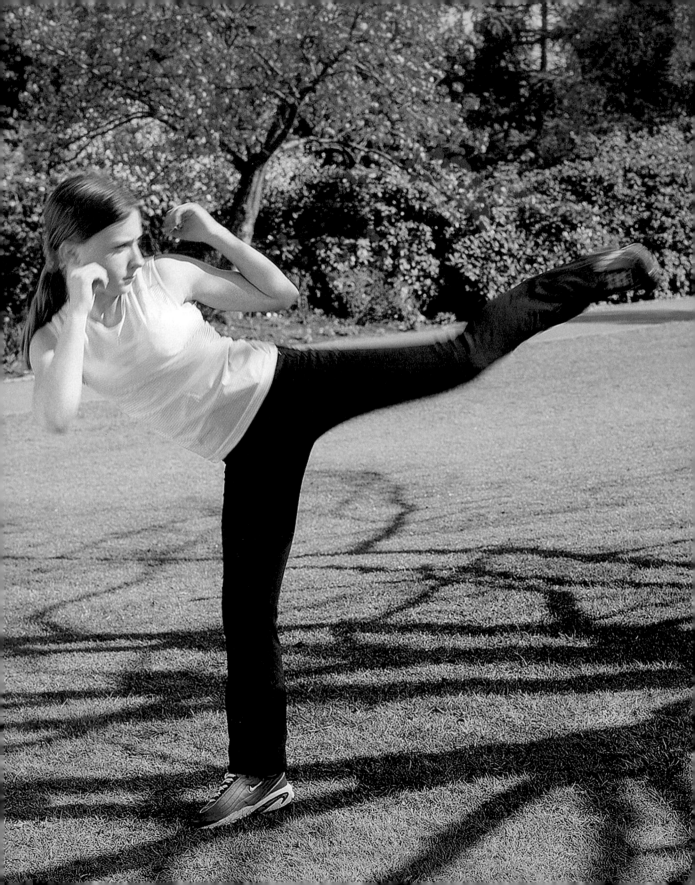

CONTENTS

Introduction — 6

1 Fat facts — 10

2 Food stuff — 18

3 Explaining exercise — 32

4 Getting started — 46

5 The warm-up and cool-down — 56

6 Kick-boxing basics — 68

The workouts — 74

7 Beginners' workout — 76

Box-a-cise class
Guest teacher: Natasha Redfern — 86

8 Intermediate workout — 92

Fat-burn circuit class
Guest teacher: Martin Ace — 104

9 Advanced workout — 112

Kick-box class
Guest teacher: Kerry-Louise Norbury and Cris Janson-Piers — 124

10 Quick workout — 128

11 Troubleshooting — 132

The next step — 152
Useful addresses — 157
Index — 158
Author's acknowledgements — 160

INTRODUCTION

I never imagined that I would become a kick-boxing practitioner, and am even more surprised to find myself writing on the subject. But, when one finds a passion, I feel it is imperative to share it.

For years I struggled with various weight problems, and this, combined with having a very low self-esteem when it came to my own body image, left me completely adrift, both mentally and physically, up to my mid-twenties. However, since discovering the world of fitness and martial arts, my life began to change for the better. It took perseverance, but my persistence paid off. Years of feeling flabby and fat, jumping on and off weighing scales like a woman possessed, faded away and I was left feeling proud of my own hard-fought abilities and fitness levels.

   I wouldn't want anyone to think that I was 'Ms Perfect' by any stretch of the imagination! I am not naturally slim or fit and I still have to work hard at it. I also have days and weeks when I really cannot find any enthusiasm for exercise or for healthy eating. But, and this is a big 'but', if I can do this anybody can. From being a flabby unfit 20-year-old, I am now a trim, healthy 36-year-old who can wear what she feels like and eat exactly what she wants. This book is a true indication not only of how I eat and exercise, but also of how I have successfully asked and guided other people to do the same.

   All you need is a little determination, some focused goals and the down-to-earth approach that not everything goes right the first time, so don't give up at the first hurdle. Only you can successfully achieve your own long-term health and fitness goals, so be your own best friend and stick with it!

   So why kick-boxing? I initially started with tae kwon do (the Korean martial art) purely by chance and have trained with kick-boxers along the way. For the purpose of this book, the benefit of kick-boxing is that it is a hybrid sport, borrowing some of its trademark moves from several martial arts. Millions of people all over the world practise it – and through it they learn how to improve their fitness, health, self-awareness, confidence and self-defence levels. For your part, this makes it one of the greatest and most interesting ways to get fit and burn fat fast. This book has taken elements from both kick-boxing and muay Thai (Thai boxing) and combined them with modern fitness knowledge. But before we look at why it is so successful in the modern fitness realm, it is important to have some understanding of the roots of both these disciplines.

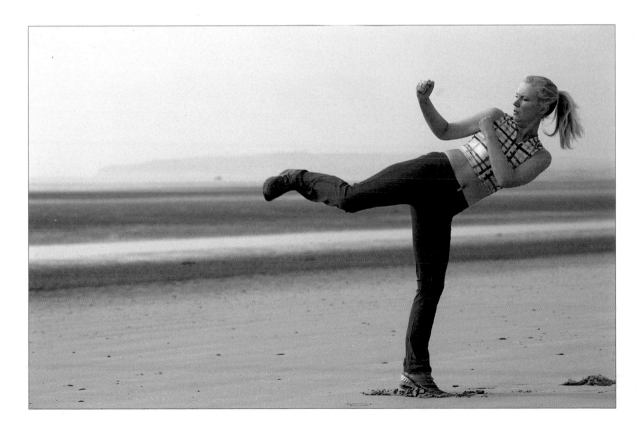

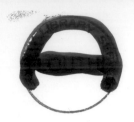

Kick-boxing

Kick-boxing is a relatively modern martial-arts system, whose syllabus was derived by combining several fighting techniques from a variety of more traditional systems, such as kyokushinkai karate, kung fu, thai boxing, tae kwon do and kyokky shinkai. Since kick-boxing is this modern hybrid martial art, it does not contain a lot of fancy footwork and doesn't have long-standing philosophies and creeds. Instead, kick-boxing offers a type of no-frills fighting that focuses on power, strength, flexibility, stamina and a blatant urge to win!

The popularity of martial arts boomed during the early 1970s, and interest was greatly increased by their emphasis on competition fighting. Chinese styles of fighting began to take on a more Westernized form in

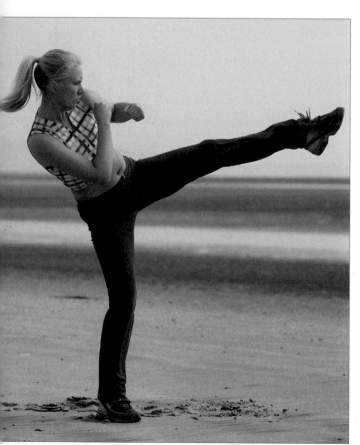

Europe, and even more so in the United States, where the first real freestyle systems were created. While many traditional martial-arts practitioners were becoming frustrated with the limitations of competition scoring, some people wished to see how effective their moves would be in a more realistic environment. Great emphasis began to be placed on specialized techniques, such as kicks and punches, being delivered with full force.

Today, kick-boxing is big business. Fights and tournaments are staged all over the Western world and many modern fitness hybrids, such as cardio kick-boxing and tae bo, have originated from it.

Thai boxing (muay Thai)

One of the most devastating fighting systems in the world, Thai boxing uses the full range of natural weapons to defeat an opponent. In the past, it was practised by warriors as part of their martial training. According to tradition, Yi Kumkam became king of Thailand by defeating his brother Fang Ken in a boxing match, thus avoiding the bloodshed of a civil war. Before the adoption of boxing gloves, Thai boxers covered their fists with hemp rope or leather thongs. It is said that ground glass was glued to the rope to make the punching more effective. However, by the 1930s boxing gloves were adopted.

The modern version has been influenced by Western boxing to some extent, improving the punching and defensive skills of the fighters, but the knee, elbow and shin techniques are all derived from the traditional art. Technically, Thai boxers are considered to be skilled in the use of the leg, knee and elbow, but, compared to Western boxers, they are poor punchers. Grappling is not permitted in the ring and there is no ground fighting. Training is very similar to that followed by Western boxers, with the addition of special methods to develop kicking power.

As with kick-boxing, muay Thai is open to most people, both male and female. It is a fast-moving and dynamic martial art, which teaches speed, power and mental agility, and increases stamina.

A winning combination

So what makes both these martial arts so effective in burning fat and helping you get fit? Simply put, it just happens to be that way. No one designed it specifically so. Over the centuries of being defined and redefined, martial arts have become an all-round holistic workout. It is the calorie-burning, sweat-inducing cardiovascular nature of throwing the various kicks and punches combined with the muscle-toning, lengthening and stretching nature of the moves that makes this a perfect workout for anyone wanting to lose body fat and tone up.

However, this workout can only touch on the essence of these martial arts. There is a whole world of kick-boxing out there, which I can only hint at here. I hope this book will be a sounding board for you and will inspire you to go out there and explore the fascinating world of martial arts.

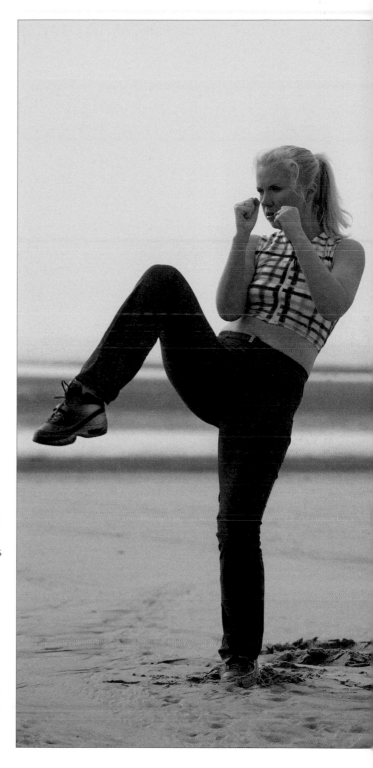

FAT FACTS

The purpose of this book is to help you lose body fat. Before we begin, it is important to arm yourself with a little information about this goal. What exactly is body fat? How much fat is 'too much'? And how can you measure your progress?

What is body fat?

Your body weight can be broken down into two components. The first is called your 'lean body mass', which comprises muscles, bones and organs. The second is your body fat.

The balance of lean body weight to body fat varies from person to person, and there is no universal ideal as our basic body shapes are determined largely by hereditary factors (more on that later, see page 15). However, there are recognized guidelines for what constitutes a healthy percentage of body fat, and our objective here is to increase the percentage of your weight that is lean body mass.

So now for the science! Body fat is the tissue in and around the muscles that is made up of fat cells. It is these fat cells that burn very slowly to sustain the body when food is scarce. However, since food in our society is rarely scarce, any excess calories we consume get stored in our bodies as fat cells just below the skin. When these cells get full, they divide to form new cells ready to be filled. A worrying fact is that these cells, once created, never go away.

Equally worrying is that half a kilogram of body fat is equivalent to only 3,800 kcals (one pound is equivalent to 3,500 kcals), which is actually not that much in terms of certain foodstuffs (grabbing a Danish pastry on the way to work every day for two weeks would be enough). It is therefore very easy to accumulate weight if we are leading a sedentary lifestyle or are not watching what we eat. However, there are ways we can keep track on what we are consuming (see Chapter Three) and we can also determine our individual daily calorie requirements by having a look at our basic metabolic rate (BMR).

Basic metabolic rate

Your basic metabolic rate is the amount of energy required to keep your resting body provided with energy for one day. One of the main influences on your BMR is your individual body composition – the more lean muscle you carry (as opposed to fat), the faster and more efficient your BMR. This is because a muscle cell, even at rest, is metabolically more active than a fat cell. Therefore, by gaining lean body mass over body fat, you will make your body much more efficient at burning calories.

How to calculate your own basic metabolic rate

While there are several things that can influence our BMR, and several different ways of calculating it, the following sum is a simple estimate that will not be far wrong for most people.

At rest, a body will use up energy at the rate of 25 kcals per kilogram of body weight per day. So, if you weigh 60 kg, your BMR is 60 x 25 = 1,500 kcals. Therefore, if you are completely sedentary, you will burn up 1,500 kcals each day. (To do this calculation in pounds, multiply your body weight by 10, then add your original weight. So, if you weigh 135 lb, your BMR = (135 x 10) + 135 = 1,485 kcals).

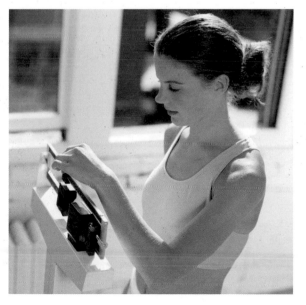

On top of this basic estimate we need to add your requirement for more calories to be consumed to fuel activity levels. This is the part of the equation that is difficult to predict, as it is not easy to measure someone's energy expenditure on the move. However, estimates that have been carried out suggest the following.

• If you have a sedentary lifestyle add 20 per cent to your daily calorie intake. A sedentary lifestyle means you have a desk-bound job and either drive or take public transport to work. Lunch breaks are spent in activities not involving any form of exercise (for example, having a quick sandwich or a visit to the pub). Your evenings are spent possibly doing some light chores or watching television.

• If you have a moderately active lifestyle add 50 per cent to your daily calorie intake. A moderately active lifestyle means you walk or cycle to work or you have an active occupation, which could involve being on your feet all day. If your job does involve a lot of sitting, you make sure you get out and about in breaks. Your evenings involve some formal exercise such as aerobic classes, swimming or a game like squash or football several times a week. Weekends, again, involve some activity like cycling, swimming or walking.

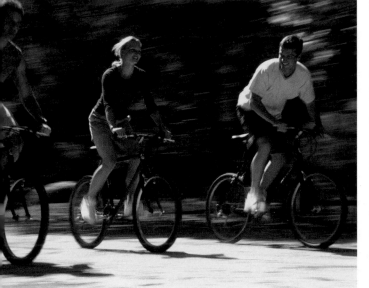

• If you have a very active lifestyle add 100 per cent to your daily calorie intake. A very active lifestyle means you have a very physical occupation, such as an exercise teacher, or you are very serious about your fitness and work out most days in addition to being very active.

As you can see, these are just guidelines. You may estimate your own activity levels to fall somewhere between these classifications – perhaps you need to add 60 or 70 per cent. If, for example, you decide your lifestyle is moderately active and you weigh 60 kg, you will burn up 1,500 kcals + 50% = 2,250 kcals per day.

Our metabolism is quite a complicated subject and we have only touched the surface of it here. However, it is enough for you to get a general idea of how body composition, exercise, food intake and general activity levels can all work together to make you a healthy fat-burning machine.

Weight versus size

It is very hard to determine by weight if you are carrying too much body fat for your age and sex. This is because muscle can weigh up to three times as much as fat. For example, two women may have exactly the same weight and be of the same height and build, yet their bodies can look completely different. One may be slender and toned while the other looks flabby and overweight. So, weighing yourself on scales can be redundant when you embark on a sensible long-term fat-loss programme.

It is quite common for people to become disillusioned a short while into an exercise programme when they find they are not actually losing any weight. In some cases, their bathroom scales may be telling them they've gained weight. This is why it's important to understand that as you get fitter and begin replacing excess body fat with lean muscle tissue, you are actually going to decrease in size. So throw away those scales, and instead watch your muscles become toned and your wobble disappear!

WHAT ABOUT CELLULITE?

Cellulite can make a sneaky appearance at any point in our lives. Despite a massive industry of skin-care creams promising to reduce or abolish this 'orange-peel' effect, cellulite is nothing more than fat. To be specific, it is the top layer of fat just underneath the skin that takes on its trademark dimpled appearance when sunlight and a natural loss of oestrogen cause the skin to thin and lose its elasticity over time. Both men and women can suffer from cellulite, but men tend to have less of it because they carry more muscle and body hair and less body fat than women do.

So, although all those products may help improve the texture of your skin, they are not going to get rid of those dimples. The only way to tackle cellulite is through exercise and eating a healthy diet.

How to measure body fat

Now you have thrown away those scales (or at least retired them), you will need to find other methods of reliable fat control. Try using a favourite article of clothing that you've outgrown; it is a great way of 'feeling' lost fat. Pick something from a point in your life where you looked and felt great (and you weren't starving yourself or over-exercising) – your goal should be an achievable and healthy size. Wear it or try it on every couple of weeks and see how it feels.

Another effective way to keep an eye on your fat level is to have its percentage measured, either at your local healthclub or with one of the following gadgets (in a range to suit any budget) that you can use at home.

All of these gadgets will come with a basic chart showing you what the sensible fat-percentage range is for your age and sex. For your general information, here are some broad figures which are accepted as an ideal healthy range.

AGE	18–39	40–59	60+
Male	8–20%	11–22%	13–25%
Female	21–33%	23–34%	24–36%

Budget

The cheapest option is to use skin-fold callipers. Most fitness clubs and personal trainers are skilled in the art of measuring body fat with callipers. Measurements are taken from four set sites on the body and added together to give you a reading of your body-fat percentage. However, this method does have its drawbacks, in that you have to be pretty skilled and experienced in order to get a correct reading, and it is impossible to do this on yourself. But for a cheap way to keep an eye on your body fat – and for a great way to get friends and family involved – they can be recommended.

Mid-range

Another option is a hand-held body-fat monitor. You simply input in your height and weight details, then the monitor sends a very mild electric current around the top half of your body and gives you a fat-percentage reading. From my regular testing of one of these monitors, I would say it is reasonably reliable. However, as it only runs a current through the top half of your body, it might not give you a completely accurate picture. But for home use, it is a great buy.

Expensive

This is a superior form of the hand-held monitor which will give you a completely accurate picture since it takes its reading from your upper and lower body. It also takes many more factors into consideration (such as your sex, age, ethnic race and how much exercise you do), which makes it, although expensive, a good investment for long-term fitness care.

WARNING
Electronic body-fat analysers must not be used by anyone who has had medical implants, such as pacemakers or defibrillators, or by anyone who is or might be pregnant. Read the manufacturer's guidelines and, if in doubt, check with your GP first.

Your basic body shape

We are all born with a pre-determined body shape which we have inherited somewhere along the line from our family's gene pool. This is simply one of those things that we have to accept. If we don't, we will spend our lives fighting a losing battle! Of course, if you have inherited your mother's stocky thighs, it is not to say that you can't do something about it (through the correct combination of exercise and diet); but they will always be part of your genetic make-up and a problem area you constantly need or want to keep an eye on.

Though the following body types are not scientifically defined, we do tend to be a combination of two of the following.

Ectomorph

Ectomorphs are tall and slim with a graceful slender neck. Usually lightly muscled with narrow shoulders, chest and hips, they will tend to have small wrists and ankles and can look quite delicate. Since they tend to have quite a naturally high metabolism, ectomorphs find it difficult to gain muscle and fat.

Mesomorph

Mesomorphs are big boned and strong looking with a muscular physique. They have broad shoulders, a narrow waist and great posture. Bearing this in mind, they can look rectangular in shape. The good news is that they find losing and gaining weight quite easy.

Endomorph

Round or soft looking, the endomorph is prone to being chubby. Broader at the hips than the shoulders and small boned, they are not naturally muscular and can carry a higher than average amount of body fat. With a slower metabolism than their counterparts, endomorphs find it hard to lose weight.

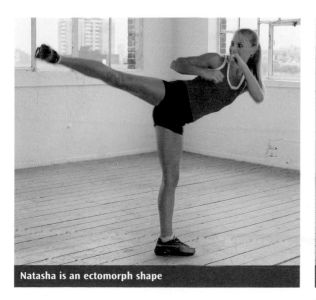

Natasha is an ectomorph shape

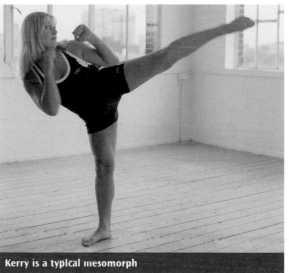

Kerry is a typical mesomorph

Body image

Before you go any further, let's have a reality check. It is all very well wanting to lose body fat, but make sure you are doing it for the right reasons.

Unfortunately a lot of people have a very negative body image and believe that 'if I only lose that extra 5 kilos then I will be completely happy with myself.' Appearance means very little compared to what's on the inside. Being thinner is not going to solve any problems surrounding a low self-esteem.

Yes, losing body fat and toning up can and should make you feel better about yourself – as long as it ends there. Almost the entire Western world is obsessed with image in one way or another, which makes it only natural that we all focus on how we look. But with the ever-increasing occurrence of eating disorders, it is incredibly important that we learn to love our bodies and respect ourselves for who we are before we embark on losing weight. Let's be clear – you don't need to have an eating disorder to have a distorted body image. Spend some time thinking over your answers to the following questions.

• **Are you preoccupied with body shape and size or are you constantly weighing yourself and feeling dissatisfied with your body?** You've taken the first step to overcoming this problem by putting away those scales – ensure they really are out of reach.

• **Do you always compare your body to others and spend a lot of time dwelling on your imperfections?** A good place to start is by stopping yourself reading fashion magazines that promote an unrealistic body type – 97 per cent of women don't look like that.

• **Do you constantly seek approval from friends and family about how you look?** Try to be your own best friend and reprogramme those negative messages others have given you with some positive ones of your own.

• **Do you frequently worry over what to wear and hiding parts of your body you dislike?** Make a list of your body parts that you do like, and think about emphasizing them instead.

• **Do you feel that worrying over your body is ruining your life and causing you to feel anxious and depressed?** This book looks at how you can nourish yourself physically, which is a vital aspect of loving your body. Take some steps towards nourishing yourself emotionally, too.

On a personal note I would like to add that prior to my career in health and fitness, most of my life was spent worrying about my weight and how I looked. With ten years of eating disorders behind me, it wasn't until the day I decided that enough was enough and I was going to attack my problems head on that I discovered the benefits of exercise. I began to eat responsibly for the first time in ten years and I followed a sensible exercise programme given to me by my local healthclub. Yes, it took a long time for my body to return to any semblance of normal but by the time it did, I had already begun to like the way I looked. Exercise and healthy eating are a way to increase your self-esteem and to love your own body – they are not a substitute for it.

Summing up

In order to lose your excess fat, you need to do three things simultaneously.

- Eat a healthy diet and cut down on excessive calories
- Exercise more
- Change your general lifestyle by adding more activity

The first two points are addressed later in the book. As for changing your basic lifestyle, all this requires is a bit of imaginative thinking and simple determination. Success in achieving and maintaining a healthy body weight is very strongly associated with an active lifestyle in which consistent exercise plays a big part. Again, like changing your daily diet, this is something that can take time to do. Try to include some form of activity (that isn't formal exercise) most days. These are only a few suggestions – the possibilities are endless.

- Always take the stairs instead of lifts or escalators.
- Leave the car at home for very short journeys like a quick trip to the local shops.
- Walk to work if possible; if not, get off the bus one or two stops earlier and walk the rest of the way.
- If you have a sedentary job, make sure you take a walk in your lunch breaks.
- Take up a leisure hobby like dancing classes or roller-skating.
- Every time you walk anywhere – no matter for how short a time – step up the pace.

Try to be as varied and as imaginative as possible. Remember, all this activity will have you burning up extra calories and helps to improve your overall fitness.

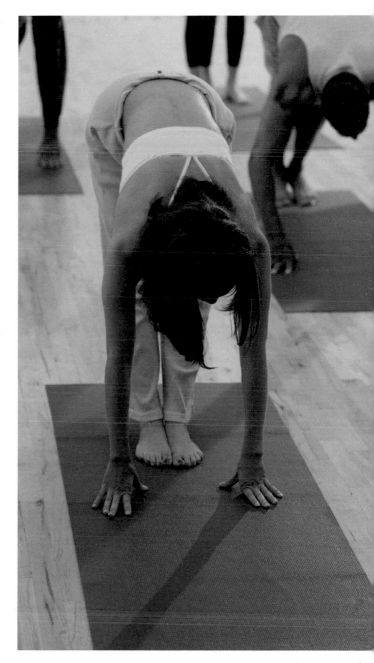

FOOD STUFF

Diets don't work – why? Because the second you start observing one is the moment you start resenting it. Even if you do manage to follow your choice of diet through to the bitter end, it is rare to find the lost weight staying off. More commonly it comes straight back on again, simply because you quickly resume your 'normal' eating habits.

A long-term view

A frighteningly common occurrence in recent years is to find yourself stuck in a vicious circle of yo-yo dieting. Too many magazines and books offer the elusive holy grail of 'lose weight quick' – which simply doesn't exist. All you end up doing is putting all the so-called 'weight' (usually more water than fat) back on and mucking up your metabolism in the process (see pages 30–31).

All these diets focus on a short-term policy of 'don't eat this for a few weeks and all your wishes will be achieved.' This is blatantly untrue, and anyone who advocates such measures should be ashamed. You should be looking at long-term goals based on what you should and can eat to stay fit, healthy and slim.

On top of all this is the physiological impact that results from constantly 'failing' at diets. I spend a lot of my working life undoing both the physiological and psychological problems that long-term yo-yo diets bring – namely, incredibly low self body image and metabolisms that don't know whether they're coming or going.

The good news is that all this can be undone with a little love and patience – from you, that is. It requires time and effort to do so, but think of the reward – how about never having to stand in front of a mirror and feel ashamed, disgruntled or worried about how you look? It is fantastic to feel positive about your body (even if it has, as every body does, a minor sag or a dimpling of cellulite) and to enjoy feeding it with healthy nutritious foods.

My philosophy is that we all know (albeit sometimes very deep down) exactly what we should and shouldn't be eating, and it is this way of thinking that has helped me give many people long-term and happy weight loss. You are also the one who knows how much you want to burn off this excess fat and what your exact motivations are. Now, with all that experience and knowledge bound up inside of you, shouldn't you be able to lose that fat once and for all?

Of course, we all need a helping hand, which is exactly what this chapter is designed to offer. Over the next few pages, I will ask you to spend time writing things down and thinking issues through. By working through these questions and exercises, you will achieve a long-term approach to healthy eating, helping you to become and stay the person you wish to be. However keen you may be to get started on any food diaries or meal plans, make sure you read this entire chapter first. There is a lot of important information to take on board, and it would probably even be worthwhile reading it through a couple of times to make sure it has all sunk in.

Why do you want to lose weight?

This may sound like a very odd question to have to answer, but it can contain a key to why you might have failed at losing weight in the past. You must be doing this for yourself and not because other people think you should. If you find your motivation is because a friend or partner has made some cutting comments about your size, and not because you actually want to lose any excess body fat, then you are unlikely to succeed. This process has to be about you and only you. You have to want to achieve your goals and you must not feel resentful about what you are about to do.

Spend some time completing the following lists. You may not be able to come up with the right answers straight away; if necessary, sleep on it and see if you agree with what you wrote in a couple of days' time. (All the way through this chapter, any examples I give are from real clients' responses, printed with their permission.)

List at least four reasons why you want to lose weight (these should be the 'cons'). For example:
- I can't fit into my summer clothes.
- I'm tired of my older sister looking better than me.
- I'm going to have to wear a swimming costume this year.
- I hate the sight of myself naked.

Now list the 'pros' to what will happen when you have lost this weight. For example:
- I can go shopping and try on clothes without feeling embarrassed.
- I will feel like I have really achieved something.
- I can feel proud of myself again.
- I can wear short-sleeved tops and a swimming costume on holiday this year.

Keeping a food diary

The next important step is to spend time writing a food diary. This will be very helpful if you want to maintain a healthy lifestyle. Writing down what you have eaten, when and why, can be a real eye-opener, even to those who think their daily diet is nearly perfect. There is always a surprising amount of unnecessary food (usually in the form of quick snacks) that can be eradicated from most people's food intake.

This process of writing down everything you eat (and how you feel before and after eating) will be the basis of your long-term healthy-eating plan. Try to spend at least five consecutive days filling in your food diary, then work through the conclusion questions to evaluate your weak areas and set yourself some goals.

It is then advisable to spend a month filling in a diary to help keep yourself on track. After the first month, you can cut this down to just one week per month, to keep you on the long-term straight and narrow. Remember, you can always go back and start again, not just with the food diary, but with your pros and cons lists, too.

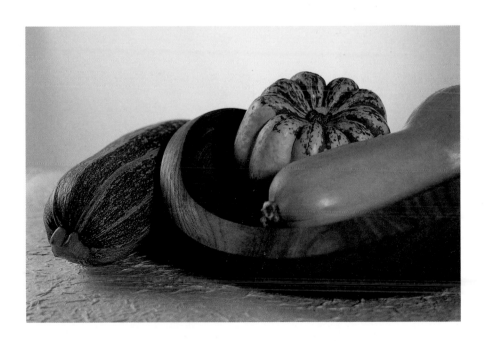

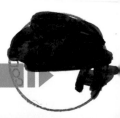

Sample food diary

Monday

Breakfast: two pieces of granary toast with butter, cup of coffee and glass of water.
Time and place: in the kitchen at 8.00 am.
Mood and feelings: woke up starving – enjoyed it very much!

Snacks and extras: one apple, four lychees and handful of cashew nuts.
Time and place: in the kitchen at 10.30 am.
Mood and feelings: pleased with myself as didn't resort to more toast.

Lunch: baked potato, beans and a small amount of mature cheddar cheese, orange juice.
Time and place: in the office at 1.00 pm.
Mood and feelings: hungry again, but pleased I hadn't picked from fridge; felt I had a bit too much though by end.

Snacks and extras: pineapple juice and more nuts.
Time and place: in the office at 3.30 pm.

Dinner: chicken sandwich with salad and mayonnaise.
Time and place: in car at 7.00 pm.
Mood and feelings: a bit resentful about having to eat my dinner in the car between work again but didn't go overboard with choice (I didn't resort to chips!)

Snacks and extras: large glass of red wine.
Time and place: at home at about 9.30 pm.
Mood and feelings: tired and bored, so this was a treat!

Notes: all in all, not a bad day – felt I had eaten reasonably healthily.

Tuesday

Breakfast: one banana and a cup of coffee from café.
Time and place: waiting for train at 8.30 am.
Mood and feelings: missed my alarm so in a huge rush and panic.

Snacks: Danish pastry and packet of crisps.

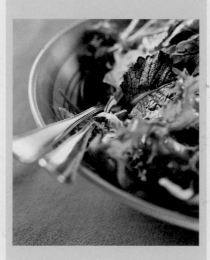

Mood and feelings: too hungry to wait for anything else and nothing decent to buy. Enjoyed while eating and do feel full but slightly guilty!

Lunch: vegetable stir-fry with brown rice, glass of water and carton of orange juice (small).
Time and place: At home at 1.00 pm.
Mood and feelings: felt I needed to eat something decent.

Dinner: three bread rolls and butter, garlic bread and king-size prawns with mayonnaise, hamburger, salad and chips; two glasses of wine, one coffee and a brandy.
Time and place: local restaurant at 8.00 pm.
Mood and feelings: I can't eat this late without small snack beforehand – I was so hungry it hurt. Was worried about eating before I went out in case I ate too much, but this is worse! MUST NOT do this again.

Notes: not such a good day. I left it too long between meals and feel that I haven't eaten a very balanced diet. However, will try and sort this out tomorrow.

Food-diary conclusions

Having spent the last few days avidly filling in your food diary, you should have noticed various weak points. Maybe not just the extra sneaky croissant you stuff down on the way to work, but also your ability to 'help' the kids finish their dinner. Spend some time looking over your diary, then read and answer the following questions.

• Did I eat normally last week or did I make an extra effort because I was keeping the diary?

• If I did make an effort, what did I do differently?

• What are my weak points that I knew about before I filled in the diary?

• Have I discovered any new weak points and, if so, what?

• What could I do to solve these weak points?

• What are my short-term goals regarding a healthier day-to-day diet?

• How can I best achieve these?

• How long am I going to give myself to achieve these goals (this can be anything from two weeks to a month)?

• What am I going to reward myself with if I achieve them?

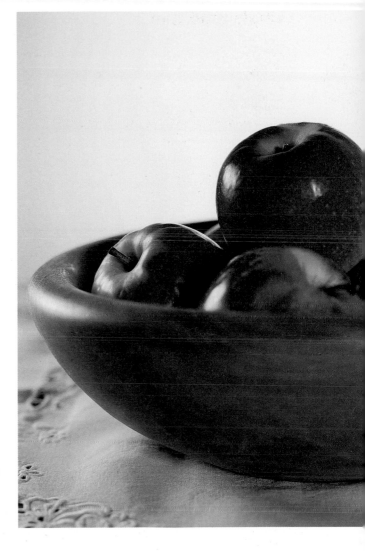

One of my clients, for example, noticed that every day, halfway through the afternoon, she couldn't resist a high-fat chocolate or cake snack. Her excuse was that at this time of day she suddenly found herself lacking in energy and starving hungry. Since she worked in an office with very little access to healthy food, and cycled to and from work, she felt that her only solution was to indulge this little whim day after day.

Unfortunately, the few pounds of excess fat she was trying to shift remained stubbornly in place. Together, we came up with a solution – she was to take a low-glycaemic snack (a slow-release source of energy) into work with her, in her case some apples and nuts as an afternoon snack. This became one of her goals – to remember to take her snack into work and to make sure she added this type of food to her weekly shopping list. She gave herself a month to achieve this, and her treat was to be a massage. The good news is that she found this much easier than she had anticipated and, eventually, that fat began to melt away again. I am not saying that this is all she had to do, but it was one of her very positive steps to achieving her long-term health and fitness goals.

What to eat

There are, of course, basic nutritional guidelines for healthy eating. It is just as important that you understand and follow these as it is for you to follow any other advice given in this chapter. As you already know, the best option for long-term health and for effective weight loss is to eat a sensible diet that combines the right quantities of the correct food stuffs.

On a daily basis, your diet should consist of: 60 per cent carbohydrate, 10 per cent protein, and 30 per cent fat. Now let's go back to basics to explain exactly what these figures mean.

Carbohydrates

Carbohydrates – or carbs – have had a very bad press recently, but really they are your best friend when it comes to sensible weight loss. There is a misconception that it is the consumption of excess carbohydrates that causes people to put on weight. In fact, we really need to make sure we eat the correct amount of carbs in order to lose fat.

No matter what form of exercise you take, the human body cannot burn fat alone. Fat can only be used for energy alongside carbohydrates. Therefore, if you are to fat-burn effectively, it is important that 60 per cent of your diet is made up of this valuable fuel source. However, there are

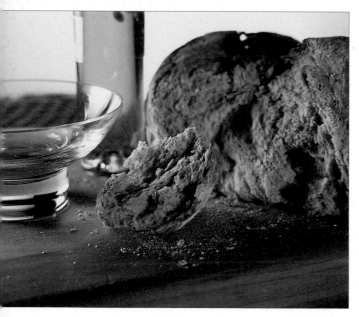

two different types of carbohydrates so make sure you are eating predominantly the right one. 'Brown' or unprocessed foods such as rice, pasta and flour are generally better than 'white', as they contain natural roughage (fibre) and goodness that is milled out in the 'processing'.

Eat more:
Complex carbohydrates (dense starchy foods such as cereals, bread, pasta, potatoes, rice and vegetables).

Eat less:
Simple carbohydrates (such as sugar, jams and sweets).

Fat

Fat is an essential part of any healthy diet and it plays many important roles within the body. To name a few: it is imperative in the uptake and storage of fat-soluble vitamins; it helps protect your internal organs; and it gives you energy.

The problem with a lot of people's fat intake is two-fold. First, an excessive intake of fat can dramatically increase the risk of ill health – obesity and coronary disease being the two main culprits. It is recommended that we consume roughly 30 per cent of our daily diet as fat, but a lot of people will find their intake veering towards the 40–45 per cent mark.

Secondly, as with carbohydrates, it is important to consume the right type of fat. Try to get your fat intake in the form of fatty fish (salmon, for example) and cold-pressed, good-quality oils for stir-frying and salads. Instead of always using butter or margarine, try olive oil instead. Try and consume the majority (if not all) of your 30 per cent daily fat intake as 'good' (unsaturated) fat.

'Bad' (saturated) fats
These come mainly from animal sources and tend to be solid at room temperature (e.g. butter, lard and cream).

'Good' (unsaturated) fats
These come mainly from plant sources and tend to be liquid at room temperature (e.g. sunflower oil or olive oil).

Protein
Proteins should be limited to 10 per cent of your daily food intake. You do need protein in order to maintain a healthy function but, like fat, a lot of people consume excessive amounts. The protein needs of most people can be satisfied by eating about 50–100 g (2–4 oz), depending on their body weight. As protein from most food sources comes in a very hydrated form, it would normally be necessary to eat something (a piece of fish, for example) weighing about 200 g (8 oz) to get 50 g (2 oz) of pure protein. However, this does mean that if you have something on your plate a few times per day that is recognizably protein, then you are probably over-consuming.

There have also been a lot of diets recently that advocate a high protein intake combined with a low carbohydrate intake. Research has shown that this advice is not only misleading but can lead to health problems. These diets can lead to fatigue due to the loss of glycogen (a vital energy source) from the muscles, but they also cause the body to break down fat differently, leading to a condition called ketosis, the side effects of which include bad breath and nausea. Excess protein is also stored in the body as fat and can cause problems with both the liver and kidneys.

Don't worry if your daily intake is a little higher than is recommended, but it is a good idea to start cutting down and replacing protein with a more useful substitute.

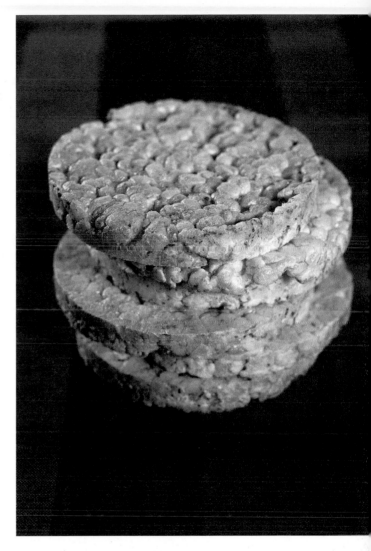

Sources of protein include:
Meat, fish, game, barley and rice, some vegetables.

Salt
Dissolved sodium (a major component of common salt) makes the blood more concentrated. To counter this, blood takes extra water out of our cells, which increases the volume of blood in the body and raises blood pressure. The RDA of salt is 3g; most of us consume three to four times that amount. Try to avoid products with added salt and don't add salt to your food in cooking or at the table.

Day-to-day eating

02

So, how do these percentages break down on a daily basis? By taking a good look at your completed food diary, you will gain some insight into exactly what you are consuming and where you need to make adjustments. A helpful way of looking at what you should be eating is the healthy-eating pyramid, which translates these general dietary guidelines into real food choices. This shows the food quantities as servings and gives a guide to how many of each you should be eating.

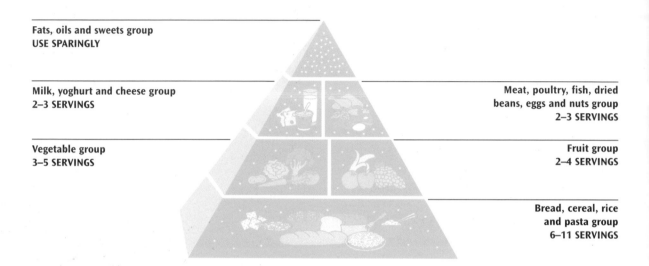

Fats, oils and sweets group
USE SPARINGLY

Milk, yoghurt and cheese group
2–3 SERVINGS

Meat, poultry, fish, dried beans, eggs and nuts group
2–3 SERVINGS

Vegetable group
3–5 SERVINGS

Fruit group
2–4 SERVINGS

Bread, cereal, rice and pasta group
6–11 SERVINGS

What constitutes a serving?

A serving is roughly 50 g (2 oz) of a particular food, but varies from one food source to another depending on factors such as water content. To give you a better idea of what this means, it translates into the following food quantities.

Bread, cereals, potatoes etc.
1 egg-sized potato
1 medium slice bread
1 small pitta or chappatti
1 bagel

3 tbsp breakfast cereal flakes
1 wholewheat cereal biscuit (Weetabix, for example)
2 tbsp cooked rice, pasta, noodles
2 tbsp uncooked oats or muesli
3 crackers or crispbreads

Fruit and vegetables
1 small bowl salad
2 tbsp vegetables
1 glass fruit juice
1 medium piece fruit (e.g. apple, pear or peach)
2 tbsp tinned fruit in natural juice
1 medium carrot or tomato
6 strawberries

Milk and dairy products
200 ml (⅓ pint) milk
1–2 eggs
small pot (130 g/5 oz) yoghurt or fromage frais
matchbox-sized (25 g/1 oz) piece hard cheese
small pot (250 g/9 oz) cottage cheese

Meat, fish and alternatives
50–100 g (2–4 oz) lean meat, poultry or oily fish
100–150 g (4–6 oz) white fish
3 tbsp pulses such as peas, beans or lentils
2 tbsp peanut butter or nuts

Ten ways to eat healthily

1. Drink lots of water

Drinking more water is one of the best things you can do for your body. Considering that we lose about 2.5 litres (4½ pints) of water a day at rest, it is no wonder most of us end up feeling sluggish by the end of the day. On top of this, we lose another couple of litres through any form of exercise (one hour's walk, for example). So it is very easy to become dehydrated.

Water will boost your energy levels and, according to one study, help your concentration. In addition, it keeps your digestive system working efficiently, helping you to metabolize fat and get rid of toxins. Some water replacement comes from our food. Fruit and vegetables, for example, have a very high water content. Ideally you should drink 2–3 litres (1 5 pints) of pure water a day, and more if you are very active. Try to take a slurp of water every 15 minutes or so. Don't wait until you are thirsty; the body's thirst response is relatively slow, so by the time you feel thirsty you are likely already to be dehydrated. Remember, also, that fizzy drinks, fruit juices and tea and coffee don't count. Some of these drinks (particularly those containing caffeine) are diuretics and can actually accelerate water loss from the body.

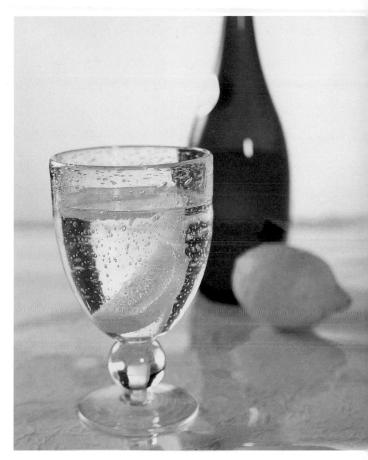

2. Think fruit and veg

Make sure you get your minimum of five portions of fruit and vegetables each day. It is not as hard as you think, and there is a great deal of scientific evidence of the benefits this can bring. Fruit and vegetables provide essential antioxidants, vitamins and minerals that the body needs to function and to fight disease. In addition, they make very handy healthy snacks.

All types of fruit and vegetables count: fresh, frozen, canned and dried. However, don't think you can just drink a carton of juice and this counts as several portions; recent guidelines show that however much juice you consume, it still only counts as one serving, so keep your intake as varied as possible. There are many ways to add extra fruit and vegetables to your diet – consider buying a blender to make your own fruit smoothies, and always add salad to

your sandwiches – you will be surprised how easy it is to eat your way through your five daily portions.

3. Eat what is in season

Eating fresh, locally grown produce is a great way to ensure you are getting the most out of your diet. The big advantage of seasonal eating is that locally grown foods are likely to be fresher than those that have been flown halfway across the world. They therefore have higher levels of vitamins, especially of vitamin C, which diminishes while fruit or vegetables are stored. Try buying from local farmers' markets, specialist shops, or you could even try to grow your own!

4. Have breakfast

The whole point of breakfast is to 'break' the overnight 'fast' and kick-start your metabolism. There is research by nutritionists at Queen Margaret College in Edinburgh that found a group of volunteers given no more dietary advice than to eat a large bowl of breakfast cereal with semi-skimmed milk every morning naturally ate less fat throughout the day and lost on average 1.5 kg (3 lb) in 12 weeks. The researchers concluded that eating breakfast could help control your weight by providing the right type of fuel for your body. By eating foodstuffs that release energy slowly, like cereal, people are less likely to experience mid-morning hunger pangs and reach for high-fat, unhealthy snacks.

5. Eat healthy snacks

Stop eating high-calorie and fat-laden snacks and you could lose up to 0.5 kg (1 lb) in just one week. You will be surprised how these empty calories add up on a daily basis. Try taking fruit to work with you, or even some nuts. Otherwise keep a container of vegetable crudities (carrots, peppers, cucumber, courgettes and cauliflower) in the fridge for whenever you get peckish.

6. Little and often

Most nutritionists recommend eating little and often. Not only is eating smaller portions (no more than two fistsful of food at any one sitting) kinder to your digestive system than huge meals, but it also helps you balance out your food intake on a even basis throughout the day, so you shouldn't experience pronounced energy highs and lows.

7. Choose well when eating out

Eating out is fun, but it can also be a minefield when it comes to eating healthily. However, it is possible (with a bit of willpower) to eat out and not completely ruin all your new-found healthy habits. Follow these tips for sensible no-guilt dining:

• Read the menu carefully and look for the healthiest options.
• Don't demolish the bread basket while perusing the menu or waiting for your food to arrive.
• Avoid food that is deep-fried, battered, or containing any cream or cheese.
• Don't be embarrassed to ask for food to be cooked

differently from what is specified on the menu. They've got the ingredients, so it is no hardship to them to cook them plainly rather than covering them with a rich sauce. Ask for your fish to be grilled or poached as opposed to fried; ask for dressing on the side when you order a salad; insist on no mayonnaise or butter with your baked potato.
• Make sure you have some vegetables and ask for them not to be covered in butter.
• If you are going to have alcohol, make sure you have a glass of water to hand. Alternate sips of alcohol and water.
• You don't have to eat it all – if you hate the idea of waste, ask for a doggy bag.
• Don't have more than two courses and make sure one contains vegetables or fruit.

8. Fish first

As I am sure you have worked out, fish is a really healthy food option. Oily fish, such as mackerel, salmon and trout, contains fats that have an important role to play in health, particularly in the prevention of heart disease. So always choose fish first, but avoid any that has been battered or covered in breadcrumbs, as this is likely to contain more unhealthy fat.

9. Eat lean

Apart from making low-fat food choices, the other major area in which you can reduce fat intake is in food preparation. Try following these tips to help you eat lean and reduce fat consumption.

• Avoid shallow- and deep-fried food. Both methods add significant quantities of fat to food and are best avoided.
• Practise low-fat cooking. There are quite a few cooking methods that do not require the addition of fat. The healthiest is steaming – this is fast, fat-free and causes minimal nutrient loss. Other ways include boiling, roasting or grilling.
• Cut back the fat. Always remove as much fat as possible prior to cooking meals such as stews and casseroles. If possible, chill meats, stews and soups after cooking so the fat rises to the top and solidifies. This can then be removed before reheating thoroughly.

• Use low-fat dairy products. Full-fat milk can be replaced with skimmed or semi-skimmed in both drinking and cooking. Mix cream with low-fat natural yoghurt or use a low-fat alternative.

• Use non-stick kitchen utensils. This helps cut down the amount of fat needed in the cooking process.

10. Portion control is important

However healthy your diet is, if you eat more calories than your body needs for energy, the excess will be stored as fat. So make sure you try and distinguish between hunger and appetite and eat sensible amounts.

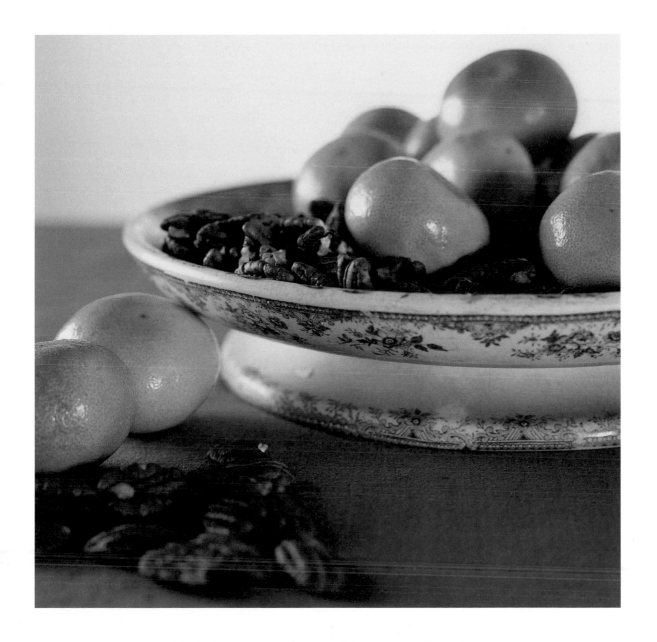

How to eat

Now we start turning all your new-found knowledge into action. You want to lose some excess body fat – just how do you do it? Put quite simply, in order to lose weight, calorie expenditure must be greater than calorie input.

Losing weight

What I hope you have gathered over these pages is that the route to successful long-term weight loss is through a gradual change in daily eating habits. The optimum sensible weight-loss rate is between 0.5–1 kg (1–2 lb) per week. Therefore, if 0.5 kg (1 lb) of fat is equivalent to 3,500 kcals (see page 11), you need to look at reducing your daily intake by 500 kcals per day in order to lose 0.5 kg (1 lb) per week.

With the inclusion of exercise, you will be burning off extra calories each day, too. So by changing what you eat, cutting down on unhealthy foodstuffs and including exercise in your daily routine, you are on the path to sensible, sustainable weight loss.

Goal-setting for food

Now you are ready to begin your personal food lists. Start by making two lists; the first one is everything you consider to be bad for you; the second is a list of foods that are good for you. From here, you can make yourself some guidelines of what you know you should and shouldn't be eating. Try to write as many different food stuffs down as possible under the following headings.

Avoid completely: chocolate and sweets, for example.
Discouraged: fast-food takeaways, for example.
Tolerated: an occasional glass of wine or beer, for example.
Welcome: fresh fruit, for example.

Now, working from the above lists, sit down and plan yourself a week's menu. Get out your cook books and rifle through; look in magazines for healthy options, or simply adapt a normal week's eating routine to include not just your dos and don'ts, but your short-term goals, too.

Your next move is to write yourself a strict shopping list and stick to it. Not only can organized shopping save you

GENERAL GUIDELINES FOR HEALTHY EATING
- Decrease fat intake to 30 per cent of total calorie intake
- Decrease intake of saturated fat
- Eat less animal protein
- Eat more complex carbohydrates
- Eat less sugar
- Eat more fruit and vegetables
- Eat more fibre-rich foods
- Decrease salt intake
- Drink more water
- Decrease intake of alcohol, fizzy drinks, coffee and tea
- Add variety to your daily diet

money, it will also help you avoid impulse purchases of banned foods.

Eat when you are hungry

This might sound silly, but a lot of people have stopped listening to their body's natural signals and mechanisms. Unfortunately, due to many years of yo-yo or non-stop dieting, you may have messed about with your hunger signals so much so that you will need to go through a process of re-learning them. So, eat when you are hungry but do not wait until you are just plain starving. However, if you do not feel hungry, do not eat – this is your body telling you that you are not in need of food.

If you have any problems with this – don't despair. There are many other people in the same boat as you. There may be reasons for not knowing when you are hungry – do you recognize any of these?

- You eat because everyone else is eating.
- You eat because it is a mealtime.
- You eat because you are sad.

- You eat because you are angry or cross.
- You eat because you are happy.
- You eat because you are bored.
- You eat because you feel fat.

Learning to discover your own natural pattern of hunger signals can take practice, time and a bit of self-focused attention. Ask yourself if you really are hungry or just in need of solace. Remember that you can re-learn these signals and become much more in tune with your body as a whole.

A little of what you fancy

Do not get too involved in eating only healthy foods. This only leads to feelings of guilt when you allow yourself to eat some 'forbidden fruit'. If you mentally banish a particular food, you will instantly begin to crave it – that is simply human nature. If you suddenly fancy something sweet, spend a few moments trying to analyse exactly what food is going to hit the target. You might decide the initial cake craving wasn't the best idea after all and what you really fancy is a sweet juicy apple. However, life is too short for you not to eat what you feel like every now and again, so if you want some chocolate, go for it – it doesn't mean you have to eat the whole bar or that you have to eat it again tomorrow. Eat it, enjoy it and then move on.

Pigging out and comfort eating

A final note – everyone has eaten either for comfort or out of pure greediness at some point in their lives. It is not the end of the world. If you are having or have had a particularly bad day and find yourself staring in an open fridge or cupboard door, stop and ask yourself, 'Is this really going to help?' You might be surprised at the answer. However, if you succumb to the temptation every once in a while, do not mentally beat yourself up over it. Pick yourself up, dust yourself down and begin afresh the next day.

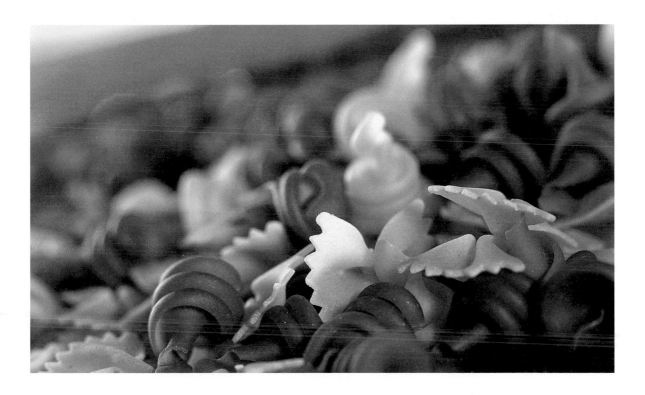

EXPLAINING EXERCISE

When buying this book you, no doubt, had a specific aim in mind. Whatever your reasons are, whether it is simply to 'burn fat' or perhaps to tone up your lower body, exercise – in particular, kick-boxing – is going to be a key tool in achieving the results you're after.

What is fitness?

Everyone has a different idea of what 'being fit' means. For some it is the ability to run for a bus without getting breathless, while for others it is being able to squeeze into a smaller size of clothing. The general consensus is that fitness enables you to go about daily tasks easily, simply and without tiring, and being able to finish the day with enough energy to run for that bus or to play a game of squash or football.

As an overall view there are four major components of physical fitness which meld together to give a broad definition and understanding of what actually being totally fit means. These are:

• Cardiovascular fitness – the efficiency of the heart, lungs and circulatory systems.
• Strength and endurance – the ability of a muscle to exert maximum force to overcome a resistance, and its ability to exert sufficient force to overcome a resistance for an extended period of time.
• Flexibility – the ability to move through your potential full range of movement.
• Motor fitness – agility, balance, coordination, power, speed and reaction time.

In order for us to have this holy grail of all-round fitness we need to work on achieving a balanced mixture of these four components. Obviously there are some times when we end up emphasizing one component more than the other, but it is important for everyone to make time for a balanced workout. Let's have a look at how these different components actually translate into workout terms.

Cardiovascular fitness

Cardiovascular fitness pertains to your body's circulatory and respiratory systems. This component of fitness may come under many guises, from aerobic training to stamina work, but the essential element remains the same. It describes our ability to take in, transport and utilize oxygen and therefore involves the efficient working of the lungs, heart and circulatory systems.

In practical terms, your cardiovascular fitness is worked on by any activity that is rhythmic in nature and uses large muscle groups to stress the cardio-respiratory system. This can mean anything that gets your whole body moving and therefore your heart, lungs and circulatory systems pumping. For example, brisk walking, jogging, running, skipping, cycling and rowing can all improve cardiovascular fitness. This 'cardio' work is a great form of exercise as it boosts your metabolism, burns calories and reduces the risk of heart disease.

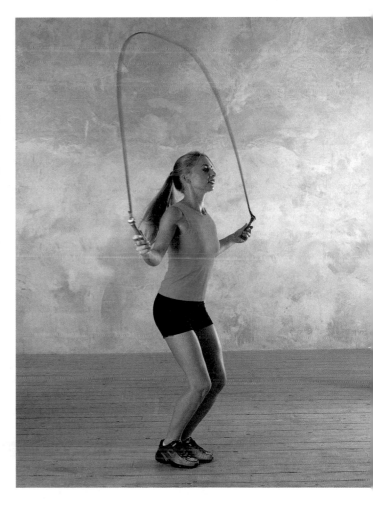

AEROBIC VERSUS ANAEROBIC

Cardiovascular fitness can be broken down into two separate components – aerobic and anaerobic. Put simply, aerobic exercise means that your muscles are using oxygen, while anaerobic means they are working without oxygen.

The balance between aerobic and anaerobic exercise depends on the intensity of the activity being done (as well as the aerobic fitness of the individual). A very simplified example would be a person doing a 20-minute fast-paced walk. They might find themselves breathing more heavily than usual but they are not out of breath. This is working aerobically. Now take the walk up a steep hill and they will find themselves out of breath by the top. This is working anaerobically. Go back to the fast walk again, and the aerobic system kicks back in. Another way to think of it is that a marathon runner works aerobically, while a sprinter works anaerobically.

What is important to note is that we can switch from working aerobically to anaerobically and back again very easily. For the purposes of this book, your kickboxing workouts should be predominantly aerobic, since you need to work out at a steady pace in order to do the kicks and punches in the workouts safely and effectively. However, there will be moments when you push yourself that bit harder and you may begin to work in an anaerobic capacity. You will find yourself getting out of breath, so need to take the pace down a notch until you begin to breathe more easily. Working at the correct percentage of your maximum heart rate (see page 40) is a good way to ensure you're working in an aerobic capacity.

Muscular strength and endurance

Unfortunately there is still a lot of distrust amongst women that this type of exercise is going give them big, bulky muscles. This type of muscle-building requires a lot of intense training every day with heavy weights, so for the average woman this is never going to transpire. What a muscular strength and endurance workout can do is help tone up your body shape, decrease flab and make you feel good!

Muscular endurance is a measure of the number of times a muscle can repeat a contraction, whereas muscular strength relates to the force (or weight) a muscle can apply in one contraction. In weight-training terms, this means high repetitions and lower weights equal an endurance programme, which is best for toning. The kick-

boxing and troubleshooting workouts in this book are ideal for this purpose. Throwing multiple kicks and punches, with your own arms and legs as the weights, is great for muscular endurance as well as being a good aerobic activity.

Flexibility

Being flexible is a very important part of your all-round fitness. A good stretching programme aims to optimize mobility and enhance the elasticity of your muscles, while maintaining the stability of your joints. There are many different types of flexibility work you can try apart from the specific workouts in this book. From differing forms of yoga and pilates to basic stretch classes, it is important to make sure this very underrated form of fitness plays a key role in

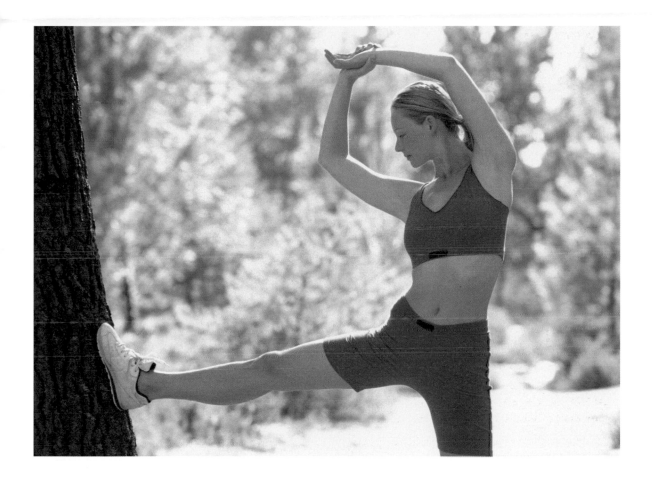

all your workouts. Being flexible aids in preventing injuries, improves your exercise technique and gets you in touch with your body.

There are two different types of stretching, both of which are used within kick-boxing. The most common is static stretching, which involves slow, sustained movements that gradually place the muscle into a lengthened position. You will use this type of stretching in your cool down when you hold yourself in the required stretch pose. The second is ballistic stretching which involves the use of bouncing or jerking movement with the aim to produce momentum generated to take the body parts concerned through a greater range of movement. This type of stretching should only be done when professionally supervised. Throwing kicks can be a

form of ballistic stretching, but I strongly recommend that you don't take any kicks or leg swings past what feels sensible and natural for your body.

Motor fitness

Agility, balance and coordination are all part of motor fitness. Every sport requires specific skills in this field, and kick-boxing is no different. A lot of people dismiss themselves as uncoordinated, but as with all the other components of fitness, these are things that can be learnt through practice and dedication. If you find it hard to kick and balance, try standing on one leg for a length of time – you will be surprised how hard this is, but also how quickly you can improve.

Why exercise?

This is not as crazy a question as you might think. There are a lot of people who cannot understand why anyone would choose to exercise. However, if you look past the cosmetic fact that regular exercise makes you look good, there are many very fundamental health reasons why you should take part in some form of fitness regime.

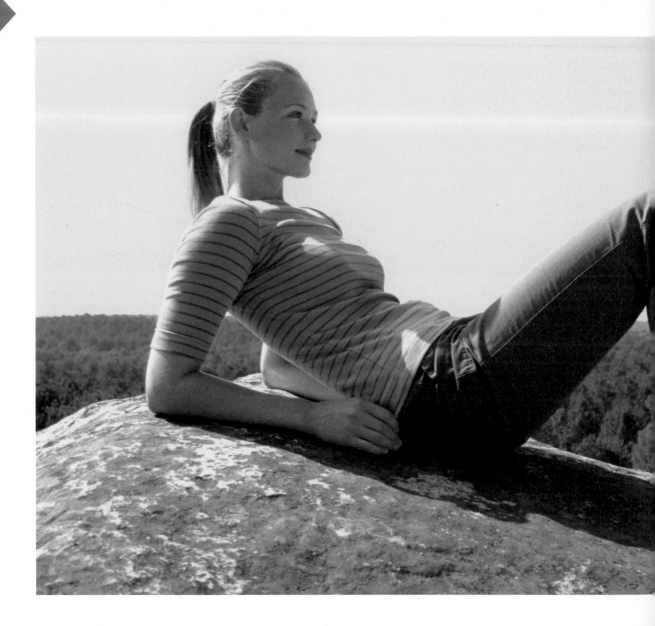

Exercise helps reduce obesity

The best way to maintain a healthy body-fat percentage is through regular exercise. Research has shown that the most successful body-fat loss in the clinically obese is when they participate in physical activity that burns 4,000 calories a week. This might sound a lot – it is equivalent to walking 65 km (40 miles) a week – but with a bit of imagination it is not impossible (see page 17 for some lifestyle activity tips).

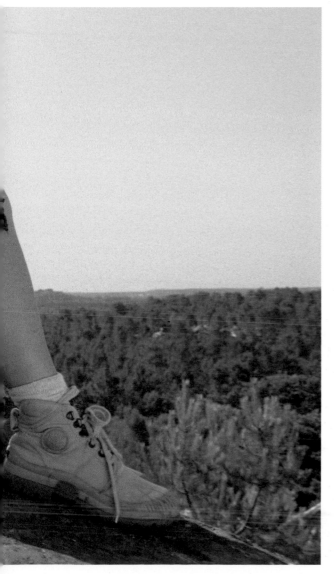

Small bouts of exercise reduce cholesterol levels

In tests, people who exercise for three 10-minute sessions a day showed greater improvements in their blood-cholesterol levels than those who exercised for half an hour in a single session.

Exercise can help prevent osteoporosis

Osteoporosis basically means 'porous bones' and is a disease in which your bone density and structural quality deteriorates, leading to fragility of the skeleton and an increased risk of fractures. One of the three factors that can help prevent its onset is exercise (the other two being hormonal activity and good nutrition). It is thought that the mechanical stresses that are put on bones during exercises can affect bone density. Therefore high-impact activities such as skipping and jogging are considered beneficial in helping combat the onset of osteoporosis, but for those not used to exercise or for the over 50s, lower impact exercise such as step aerobics or intermittent jogging is more appropriate.

Exercise improves glucose intolerance

Regular exercise and physical activity can improve blood-glucose regulation and reduce the need for diabetic medication. If you are diabetic, it is important to consult your doctor before undertaking any exercise.

Regular exercise reduces blood pressure

Studies show that regular exercise reduces blood pressure. However, if you are at all concerned about your blood pressure or do not know your blood pressure then you must check with your doctor before taking any exercise.

Exercise makes you feel good

Not only has it been shown that exercise can improve your mood, but it has also been found to be effective in combating depression. In addition, it can increase your self-confidence by helping you get in tune with your body.

How exercise works

There is no hidden magic to exercise – if you follow the basic principles you are going to get results – it really is that easy and logical!

The overload principle

In order to make improvements in fitness, your body must do more than it can comfortably manage. When this happens, the heart, lungs, circulatory system and muscles are challenged, and they have to overcome the demand placed upon them. Since they are forced to adapt, they get stronger, so the next time they can respond to the overload more easily. By this principle, you can start your exercise programme on day one, only able to manage just a brisk walk, but if you keep stressing your body by asking it to do a little more each time, by day 30 you would be able to manage a slow jog.

Progression principle – FITTA

A lot of people new to fitness can fall into the over-enthusiastic category. Though this type of positive thought has its benefits, it can often lead to individuals doing too much, too soon, which results in tired muscles, pain and a generally low morale, leading to them giving up all together.

What everyone new to exercise always wants to know is – when will I see results? Unfortunately this is a very hard question to answer, since it depends on the individual and their reaction to the exercise involved. However, there is a simple principle which, if followed, is guaranteed to bring sensible long-term results. This is called FITTA.

Frequency

This refers to the number of times you exercise over the course of the week. To get the best out of your workouts, modern guidelines suggest you work out at least three times a week in order to be see some steady long-term improvements.

Intensity

The degree of effort you need to put into your exercise is also important. If, for example, the workout suggests you do a fast jog and all you muster is a steady walk, then you wouldn't be working out at a high enough intensity for you to be getting anything out of the workout.

Time

This is about the length and duration of each exercise period. Simple – if the workout is meant to take 30 minutes and you manage to cut it down to 5 minutes then the only person you are cheating is yourself.

Type

It is necessary to vary the type of exercise undertaken (see specificity below, and cross training, page 52–54). While kick-boxing is going to be your main type of exercise, it is important to complement this with the troubleshooting workouts (see pages 132–151) and other cardio options.

Adherence

This means that you have to stick to the programme to get results! If you don't keep exercising, your body will naturally slow down and work less efficiently – and all your hard-earned fitness will go to waste. On page 55 you will find long-term exercise suggestions for all levels. In order for this (and other) workouts to be successful, you need to stick to these plans.

Specificity

The benefits of your exercise workouts will be a result in the particular demands you place on your body. We can all think of people who we consider fit – maybe we see them out running every morning, charging ahead while their partner lags along behind. However, put the same people in a kick-boxing class or in a swimming pool, and we may find them getting out of breath or having to rest after only a very short time.

What this shows is that in order to achieve a specific result, we need to train with that in mind. So, if you want to lose fat and tone up your body, the workouts in this book are perfect for you. But if you wish to run a marathon, then you need to be doing some running instead. Once again, it is very important to think about cross training (see page 52–54) to prevent your body getting into the habit of doing the same thing week in and week out. Everybody needs variety, not least to combat the boredom factor, but also to make sure we keep our body on its fitness toes.

Rest and recovery

This is where the novice exerciser often goes wrong. In your keenness to get results, don't overlook the fact that your body needs time to recuperate after bouts of exercise. Just as your body needs to re-charge its batteries every day with a good night's sleep, so too do your muscles, so try do your main workouts every other day in order to get optimum benefits.

A note about sweating!

We all sweat, but at different points in our workouts. A lot of people are embarrassed because they sweat so readily, but they shouldn't be – it is just the way they are made. In fact, the fitter you are, the more quickly you are likely to sweat – think of it as having a very efficient central-heating system. However, this is not set in stone and some people never seem to muster more than a gentle glow.

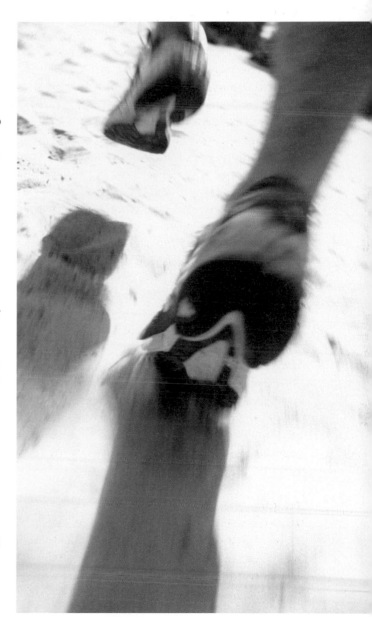

When shouldn't you exercise?

Though a lot of us seem to spend time trying to fit exercise into our hectic lives, there are times when we should be doing completely the opposite – absolutely nothing. No doubt this might come as a shock to some (and a relief to others) but there are points in our lives when taking it easy does us the power of good. Before you throw out your trainers for good, I would like to point out that this should be restricted to the following reasons:

03

• 'I am just too tired.' Sometimes this is a valid excuse. There are days when it will do you the power of good to give yourself permission to have a day off your fitness programme. Just make sure you eat healthily, do not mentally punish yourself – and enjoy it.

• 'It's only a touch of flu, I can still exercise.' No you can't. If you are not well, you shouldn't be exercising at all, even if it is just a cold. All you doing is prolonging your illness and hindering a proper return to exercise.

• 'I am nearly over it.' If you have been ill for a couple of weeks or even a couple of days, don't go rushing back to your normal exercise routine. Make sure you have recuperated first and start slowly. Going back into exercise before you are ready sets back your recovery.

• 'It was only a pulled muscle.' Whatever your injury was, make sure it is thoroughly healed before you get back into training. What may have been a simple injury at first can be worsened by your well-meaning attempts to 'loosen it up'. If you are unsure always seek advice from a physiotherapist or an osteopath.

• 'I only had a couple of drinks.' If you have any form of hangover, please think twice before you go rushing into your early-morning workout. Take time to consider how alcohol can severely dehydrate you. Have you drunk enough water to balance out its effects? Are you still under the influence? Alcohol can be slow to work its way out of your system. Finally, when did you last eat? Sometimes the idea of eating on a hangover is the last thing you want to do. So, if you haven't eaten enough to be training – don't do it.

• 'What if I am pregnant?' If you think you are pregnant, then stop kick-boxing until you know for sure. You can exercise throughout your pregnancy provided your doctor or midwife says you can, and you feel happy doing so, but the emphasis and the type of exercise need to change.

Setting the pace

As each workout is designed to get you hot, perspiring and burning calories, it is important to make the most of your time doing it. By this I mean you need to be working hard enough for you to see results, but not so hard that you start to work anaerobically. In order to do this, you need to keep track of your heart rate to make sure you are working in the correct zone for your age and fitness level.

Maximum heart rate

To burn fat efficiently, you need to work within your optimum training zone, which is between 70 and 90 per cent of your maximum heart rate (MHR). In order to keep a check on this, you need to learn how to calculate it. Though this might seem a bit complicated to begin with, it won't be long before it is second nature and you will be able to recognize instinctively if you are exercising in the right zone.

To work out your own MHR, all you need to do is subtract your age from 220. So a 35-year-old has an MHR of 185 (220-35=185) beats per minute (bpm). From here, with the aid of a calculator, you can work out the MHR percentage you are required to work at. For example, if the workout suggests you work at 80 per cent of your MHR, then the heart beats per minute for a 35-year-old should be 148 bpm. This figure of 148 represents the heart rate you should be aiming for throughout the main body of the workout; obviously it is very hard to be exact, but this is your ball-park figure.

For ease, the approximate figures for percentages of MHR are given in the table opposite. Each of the workouts in this book will give you some guidelines as to which level of your MHR you should be working at. Do remember that if the workout asks you to work at a certain MHR and you find yourself working too high, then you need to slow down (and vice versa). For example, if in the beginners' workout you need to be working at 134 bpm (age 26–30 at 70 per cent MHR) and your heart rate is up at 160 bpm, then you need slow down the intensity.

Here are three good ways to keep track of your heart rate while exercising.

Rate of perceived exertion (RPE)

When you have become familiar with how your body responds to exercise, the RPE scale on the following page is a quick and simple way of checking how hard you are working. The scale itself is based on your body's physical response to exertion. It runs from one to ten: at one you are at rest, while at ten you are working at your hardest.

This form of monitoring does rely heavily on your own judgement, so it can be tempting to cheat by convincing yourself you are working harder than you actually are. But remember, it is only yourself you are cheating!

APPROXIMATE PERCENTAGES OF MHR FOR AGES 18–55					
Age (years)	70%	75%	80%	85%	90%
18–25	139	149	159	169	179
26–30	134	144	153	163	172
31–36	130	140	149	158	168
37–42	126	135	144	153	162
43–50	121	129	138	147	155
51–55	116	124	133	141	149

Heart rate monitors

This is the easiest (and most accurate) way to monitor your heart rate. This piece of equipment can do all the work for you and is relatively inexpensive. It consists of a strap around your chest that monitors your heart rate and sends a signal to a watch-like device on your wrist, providing a continuous and consistently accurate reading. You can buy these monitors from most department stores and sports shops, but be aware that there are a number of 'extras' which can bump up the cost. Do not be forced into spending your life savings on one of these – you really only need the most basic model.

Pulse taking

Taking your pulse is an accurate way of checking your heart rate, the only disadvantages being that you have to stop to do it and it can be quite tricky to the inexperienced. However, with a bit of practice, it is relatively foolproof. To take your pulse, find your pulse point at your wrist; follow the line of your thumb, then place two fingers (not your thumb) about 2 cm (1 in) below your wrist joint. Count for 15 seconds, then multiply by four to get your beats per minute (bpm).

RPE Scale		
Level	Activity level	Heart rate
1	at rest	non-exercise heart rate
2	low-level activity, such as standing	non-exercise heart rate
3	light exertion, such as gentle walking	non-exercise heart rate
4	purposeful walking	non-exercise heart rate
5	brisk walking	non-exercise heart rate
6	medium/fast pace walking	60% MHR
7	breathing becomes more difficult, you feel hotter	70% MHR
8	breathing heavy, beginning to sweat, can just converse	80% MHR
9	sweating, difficult to hold conversation	90% MHR
10	maximum effort, hard to maintain for long	maximum heart rate

Explaining your workout

As you now can see, an effective fitness programme needs to incorporate cardiovascular work, resistance training (muscular strength and endurance) and stretching. These are all important factors for fat loss, too, but the balance needs to be correct. Your workouts within this book aim to reduce the amount of fat on your body and to tone the shape of your muscles, giving you a firmer figure. This, in turn, will also give you the long-term benefits of making you into a lean, mean, fat-burning machine. As a basic overview, each of your workouts should break down as follows:

Warm-up

The warm-up is designed to get you both mentally and physically prepared for the workout to come. For this you are going to use a series of different exercises that slowly build up in intensity. By doing this, you are bringing your heart rate up slowly and safely whilst letting all the muscle groups warm up and mobilize.

Kick-boxing routine interspersed with cardio breaks

The kick-boxing routine is effective on two counts: it is aerobic, so you are working your cardiovascular system in order to burn calories and improve the capabilities of your heart and lungs; in addition, it is a muscular endurance workout, toning the major muscle groups.

The cardio breaks (skipping or jogging, for example) give your muscles a break from their endurance workout and provide you with an opportunity to keep an eye on your heart rate. If you find it is hard to keep your heart rate up in the correct zone during the kick-boxing, you can up the intensity of your cardio break, thereby increasing your heart rate. You could do this by increasing the speed of your skipping or running around a bit faster than normal. On the other hand, if you find yourself working too hard (getting slightly out of breath or your heart rate continually getting too high), you can use the break to take your heart rate down slightly – try doing fast-paced marching instead of running or skipping.

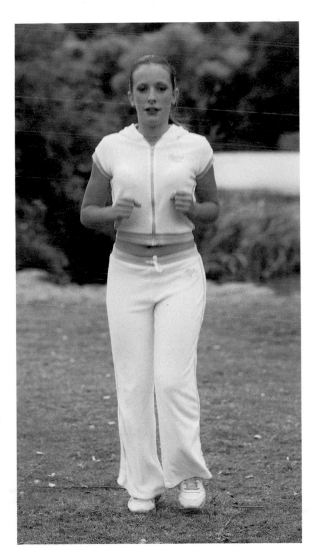

Cool down

The cool down is there to help you take your heart rate down safely by using exercises that decrease in intensity of activity slowly. The idea is to take your working heart rate back down towards your resting heart rate (what you started with before you did any exercise at all).

Troubleshooting workout (if desired)

On top of working out in your correct MHR zone, you need to add some resistance work in the form of trouble-shooting. This is the muscular strength and endurance part of your workout, designed to target various common trouble spots. You choose the areas you want to work on.

Initially, you may be getting sufficient muscle-toning benefit from simply following the kick-boxing workouts. But as time progresses (and your body adapts) you will need to move on and change your workouts slightly to include some different resistance work. Recent research has shown that it is this type of exercise – a mixture of cardiovascular work and resistance training (either body toning or strengthening) – that is most effective at producing fat loss.

Stretch

This is the last part of every workout, but it is just as important as the rest. Use this time to relax and stretch out every muscle group used to ensure that you maintain all-round flexibility.

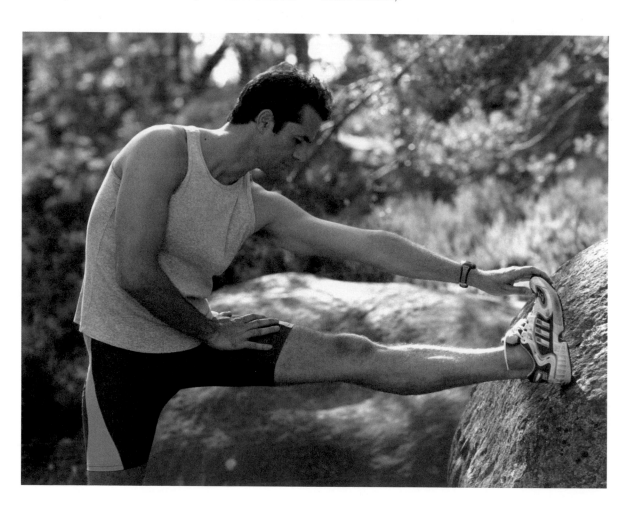

TRAINING DIARY

Your training diary is one of the most important tools you can use for long-term success in a fitness programme. In much the same way as you write down your daily diet (see page 22), revealing all your ups and downs, a training diary will show you how often you have been exercising and can help keep you motivated. It is also a great way to plan ahead (in conjunction with your social and work commitments) exactly what exercise you wish to do and when.

You can buy special training diaries from sports shops, but a normal one will do the job just as well. Make sure you record daily whether you have done any exercise (and general activity), what is was and how long you did it for. You can also record how you felt (any aches or pains, whether you found it particularly hard work or easier than before) or even if you meant to exercise and didn't!

As with your food diary, spend some time looking back over it. You will often find a pattern emerging for good and bad days – for instance, if you find that early-morning exercising isn't working out for you, you might want to try shifting your workouts to the late afternoon or evening.

Relax and recuperate

Finally, there are two more things you need to do as part of your exercise programme – relax (with the stretching) and recuperate (take time off). As you have seen, both of these components are essential to a successful exercise programme, so make the most of them.

There are plenty of things you can be doing on your rest days. Rest doesn't mean you have to do absolutely nothing. As part of the plan is to raise your metabolic rate, it is a good idea to get some of your much-needed activity in on these days (see page 17) or, if this all feels too much, spend your downtime taking up a relaxing hobby such as tai chi or meditation – both of which will do wonders to enhance your overall well-being.

CHAPTER FOUR

GETTING STARTED

It is all very well deciding that you want to get fit and lose some excess body fat, but what happens next? A lot of people who take up exercise find themselves enthusiastically pursuing their goal for the first few weeks and then tailing off. This is usually down to a lack of pre-planning and can be easily remedied. Like anything you do, it is vital to plan your exercise routine ahead; find your motivation, and be determined to stick at it. Preparation is always half the battle, so make sure you work through this chapter thoroughly before progressing onto the workouts later in the book.

Where to kick-box

All you need is adequate space. By this I mean somewhere you can stretch out a kick without fear of knocking over anything precious or hurting yourself on a piece of furniture. Exactly where you choose is completely up to you. I personally enjoy working out in the great outdoors when the weather permits. There is nothing like the freedom of open space and fresh air in your lungs. It needn't be anywhere where you are likely to draw a small crowd – your back garden or terrace will do. However, most people prefer the privacy of their own homes, and with a bit of furniture rearrangement, the workouts in this book are designed with this in mind.

Choose a room that is adequately ventilated and has enough space for you to move around in. If you have nosy pets, children or housemates, then use a room where you can lock the door or stick up a 'do not disturb' sign. Also, it is often useful to have a full-length mirror for checking your technique and some motivating music to listen to. Finally, remember to keep a bottle of water to hand to keep yourself hydrated throughout.

What to wear

Your most important piece of clothing, whatever form of exercise you are doing, is your trainers. If you haven't bought a pair in years, now is the time to invest in some new ones. You don't have to spend a fortune. The best bet is to opt for a cross-trainer, designed for use in studio-based classes or for gym work, rather than a running shoe. You need good cushioning in the heel and the ball of your foot to lessen impact when you jump, plus a design that offers lateral stability (support for the sides of the feet) to help you balance. Buy trainers at the end of the day when your feet are at their largest and wear the type of socks you intend to work out in. You may find you need the next size up from your normal shoe size, so make sure you ask to try on lots of different pairs of various sizes and makes, as different manufacturers' styles suit different foot shapes.

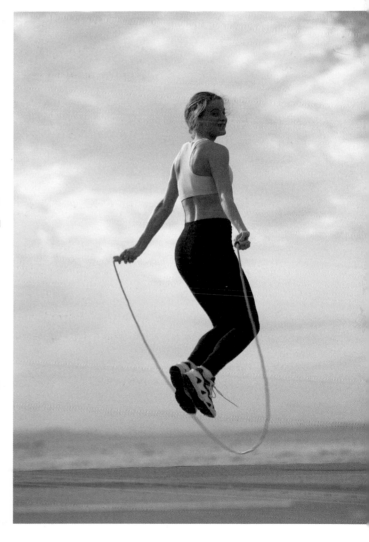

Clothes-wise, it's best to wear what you feel comfortable in and what allows you a decent range of motion. Most of the big sportswear brands produce ranges with loose-fitting trousers and tops – look for clothes made out of fabrics that allow you to sweat, whether they are cotton or specially developed manmade fibres such as Gortex. It's a good idea to dress in layers so you can peel off clothes as you warm up and replace them as you cool down.

Basic equipment

You don't need any equipment to get started, but you will find the following three items useful.

Exercise mat

There are many different mats available to buy, in a wide price range. The main points to think about are thickness and ease of care. If you are planning on doing most of your floor-based exercise on a carpet, you needn't worry about how thick the mat is – the carpet or rug can do most of the cushioning for you. However, if you are going to be working out either outdoors or on floorboards, then it is advisable to spend a little extra on a thicker mat. Look for a mat that is easy to clean (this is usually done by just washing it down with a damp cloth), since you will sweat into it. If you don't have a mat, a thick towel or rug is a good substitute.

Skipping rope

Ropes come in many forms and your choice is really a matter of personal preference. You can go with one made of either plastic or rope, but make sure that the length is adjustable as it is important the rope is the correct length for your height. To check the length, stand on the middle of the rope, with your feet hip-width apart, and pull the handles upwards until the rope is taut. The handles should be in your mid-chest region, just under the line of your armpits. Most ropes come with instructions on how to shorten them. If yours doesn't, try unscrewing the handles and pulling the rope through. If you don't manage to get hold of a skipping rope, you can try 'virtual skipping' (imagining you are jumping over a rope); but a rope is a worthwhile piece of equipment to invest in.

Hand weights

Hand weights can be also bought in many guises, from chrome-plated to foam-covered; again, it is a matter of personal choice. I prefer chrome because, as with the mats, they are going to have sweaty hands holding them and are easy to wipe clean. However, some people prefer the feeling of the softer foam-covered weights or the coloured plastic ones. If you buy two different weights – I suggest a 2.25-kg (5-lb) and a 4.5-kg (10-lb) set – these will see you through all the exercises in this book. You can use various substitutes for hand weights – try filling small, empty water bottles with sand or small stones.

Resistance bands

Made out of rubber, these are available in various strengths, usually differentiated by colour, although the colour coding varies from manufacturer to manufacturer. The idea is that you wrap them round your foot or hand and push against them (see pages 133–4). Resistance bands are a very cheap, portable and effective way of adding resistance to your workout.

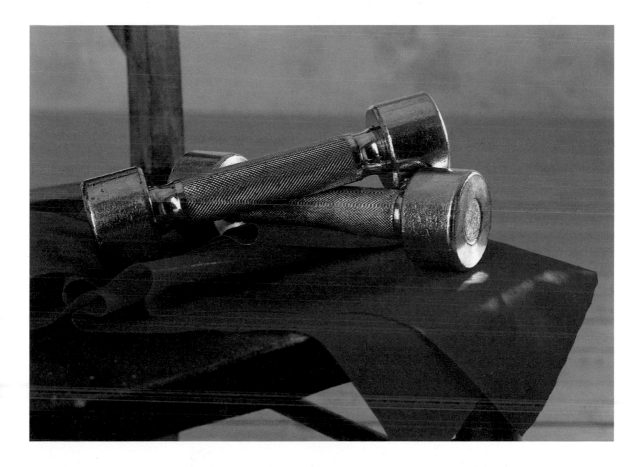

Questionnaires – are you fit to get fit?

Do you need to see a doctor?

It is always sensible to consult your medical practitioner if you have any doubts about starting this or any other exercise programme. Work through the following checklist and, if you answer 'yes' to any following questions, then you must consult a doctor before beginning any of the workouts or exercises contained in this book.

• Have you ever been diagnosed with a heart condition, or is there a history of heart disease in the family?
• Are you more than 20 kg (42 lb) overweight?
• Do you have high blood pressure or do you not know your blood pressure?
• Are you asthmatic or do you have a history of breathing problems?

• Are you diabetic?
• Are you pregnant or trying to become pregnant?
• Have you recently given birth?
• Have you had surgery in the last six weeks?
• Have you recently experienced chest pain during physical activity?
• Have you ever been advised by a doctor to avoid exercise?

...or a physiotherapist?

'Prevention is better than cure' is an adage that is especially true in the world of exercise. There is no point starting an exercise programme with all the good intentions in the world only to find yourself suffering from a pre-existing injury (perhaps one you weren't even aware of), which can then put you out of action for a considerable amount of time.

Unfortunately, modern life forces our bodies into physical situations for which they were not designed, such as sitting hunched over a computer or steering wheel for hours at a time, or simply carrying the same heavy bag on the same beleaguered shoulder day in and day out.

A lot of people consult physiotherapists (or related professionals, such as osteopaths and chiropractors) as a matter of course. If you have any doubts or answer 'yes' to any of the following questions, I strongly advise you to do the same.

• Do you suffer from knee pain (when walking downstairs, for example)?
• Have you ever had shin splints?
• Do you suffer from lower back problems?
• Do you suffer regular twinges in your shoulders or upper back muscles?
• Have you ever been told not to exercise for any length of time by a relevant professional (such as a physiotherapist)?
• Do you have bunions or other foot problems?
• Have you ever fractured or broken any bones?
• Have you ever had surgery on a joint or ligaments?

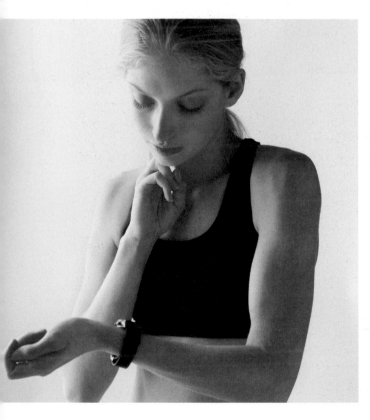

Assessing your fitness level

These are very simple fitness tests designed for you to do at home. They are here as a general guideline for you to get a better idea of the demands you should be making on your body. If you would like a more in-depth fitness assessment, then most healthclubs and gyms will offer you a professional service and guide to your own individual fitness level.

1. The hip-to-waist ratio

This test assesses your body shape and fat distribution. Measure your hips, then measure your waist. Divide your waist measurement by your hip measurement and score as follows.

	Score
WOMEN:	
above 0.86	1
0.71–0.85	2
below 0.7	3
MEN:	
above 0.95	1
0.81–0.94	2
below 0.8	3

2. The one-minute sit-up test

This test is to assess your strength in general, and the postural strength of your stomach muscles in particular. Lie on your back on the floor with your knees bent and your feet flat on the floor. Your spine should be in a neutral position and your abdominal muscles tight. Place your fingers at the sides of your head, gently cupping your ears with your hands and allowing your elbows to fall naturally out to the side. Keeping a space between your chin and your chest and breathing out, lift up your shoulder blades, shoulders and then head. Return to the ground under control.

Perform as many sit-ups as you can in one minute. It doesn't matter too much if you have to stop and start, as long as you keep a good technique throughout. Score as follows.

	Score
24 or below	1
25–45	2
46 or more	3

3. The step test

This is a test of your cardiovascular fitness (see page 33). Use a step or a chair that is 40 cm (16 in) high. Stand facing the step or chair and step up with one foot, placing the whole foot flat on the step. Keep your back straight and abdominals tight. Now step up with the other foot, so both feet are flat on the step. Step down with your leading foot, then with your second foot.

Repeat these step-ups at a rate of 30 per minute for 3 minutes. Stop, then take your pulse (see page 42) for 15 seconds. Multiply this figure by 4 and score as follows.

	Score
WOMEN:	
167 or more	1
141–166	2
140 and below	3
MEN:	
157 or more	1
131–156	2
130 and below	3

Working out your scores

Tot up your scores for exercises 1, 2 and 3. Your total will give you an indicator of your fitness level. If you scored 5 or less, then you should start working out using just the beginner-level workout until you feel ready to progress to the next level. If you scored 6 or more, then you could begin working out with the beginner and intermediate-level workouts. However, I advise starting with only the beginner-level workout for the first week and moving on when you feel confident enough to do so.

Your cross-training workout

Since variety is the key to a successful long-term workout routine, I strongly recommend you use the exercise programmes given in this book as part of an overall cross-training workout. Follow the weekly workout routines by planning ahead, writing down your programme in a diary and then making sure you stick to it.

However great it is to learn a new skill, there will come a time when your enthusiasm begins to wane. This is when cross training really comes into its own. Its benefits are multiple: it provides interest and variety; it reduces the risk of injury; and, as no one activity provides full fitness benefits, a varied workout is the perfect choice. Not only that, but cross training also helps expose you to the manifold joys of exercising!

So, how can cross training reduce the risk of injury? Any one activity involves the same repetitive action, which is continually channelled through a certain part of the body. With running, for example, every footfall can send a shock through the feet, legs and spine equivalent to three times the runner's weight. By varying your aerobic workout to include lower-impact activities that will still improve your cardiovascular system, you develop a sensible, injury-free way of training.

Here are some ideas for you to choose from.

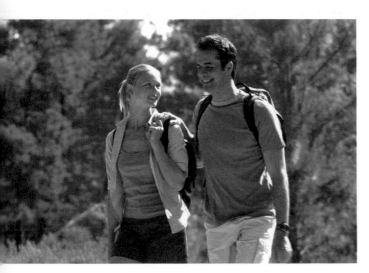

WHAT IS CROSS TRAINING?
Cross training is the practice of training in more than one sport. It is a strategy used by informed exercisers and professional athletes to organize their workouts and fitness activities, with the aim of providing as much variety and challenge as they need to stay on track in achieving their fitness goals in a safe, interesting and satisfying way.

Walking

This is one of simplest and cheapest ways to get and keep fit. All you need is your body, a decent pair of shoes and some motivation. The American Journal of Clinical Nutrition recently published a report that looked at people who had sustained long-term weight loss; unsurprisingly, 94 per cent of them had done this by increasing their level of exercise, but the relevant point is that the majority of these had done so through walking. There are lots of different types of walking, from speed walking to rambling through the countryside, but do be aware that a wander down to the local shops will not have quite the same effect as a brisk walk!

Research has now shown the number of steps you should take each day to achieve specific activity goals: 4,000 steps a day will improve your health; 7,000 will increase your fitness level; while 10,000 can contribute to weight loss. What is so good about this is that you don't have to do it in one hit; you can accumulate your daily step total as you go about your normal activities. To keep track, you'll need a pedometer (a simple device that measures your individual stride count) – and remember to keep it brisk.

Running

Moving on from walking is another simple form of exercise – running. Though it may not be everybody's idea of fun, it is a great and easy way to improve your cardiovascular system and burn calories. As with walking, all you need is a decent pair of shoes and enough motivation to get (and keep) you going.

04

The main difference between this and walking is that running is a high-impact activity, with the impact working its way through your legs and back, making it unsuitable for some people. Check with your doctor or personal trainer if you have any qualms over your ability to run.

The key to successful running is to start slowly and build up, so don't be put off by all those people you see charging past you in the street or park. Begin by speed walking on a regular basis, then start to intersperse this with short, slow jogs – you will soon find you can work up to a continuous run. If you feel that this could be a lonely affair, check out local sports shops or health clubs for running clubs in your area. These normally meet once a week and will cater for every fitness level.

Swimming

Swimming is a great way to improve your cardiovascular fitness, and has the added benefit of working your entire body while being completely non-impact. Water acts as a giant cushion for the body and is kind to vulnerable joints and tendons, which makes it a great medium in which to exercise if you are overweight, pregnant or suffer from joint problems.

Even if you are not a great swimmer, you needn't dismiss this as an option. There are many adult swimming classes available, both for those who simply have never learned to swim properly and for nervous or 'rusty' swimmers. Either way, you will improve your water skills. In addition, most pools and health clubs offer aqua-aerobic classes that cater for all levels.

Cycling

Not only is cycling a great way to get and keep fit, it is also an enjoyable leisure activity and a simple, environmentally friendly way to get to and from work and play. Cycling is a low-impact cardiovascular activity and, like many of the other cross-training options, comes in many guises.

You could try any of the various spinning classes available in local gyms. These involve an instructor leading a class on stationary bikes through a simulated cycling workout. With the added benefit of music and the other participants, you will get a great workout specifically geared to your fitness

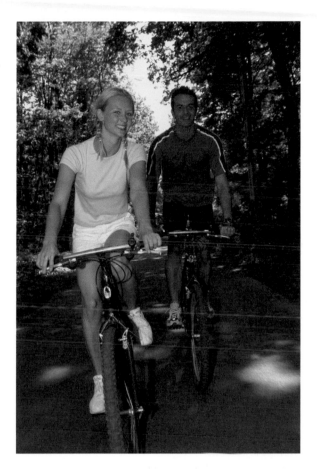

level. Otherwise, you can dust down your old bike (making sure you get it thoroughly serviced by a professional) and take to the great outdoors. As an added bonus, according to the British Medical Association, cycling keeps you young. A recent study discovered that regular cyclists have fitness levels equivalent to non-cyclists 10 years their junior!

Racket sports

If you are more of a social exerciser, then one of these could be the game for you. Squash, tennis and badminton can be played all year round and are an interesting way to improve your fitness – including your motor fitness (see page 35). Since they are 'stop and start' sports, they place demands on both your aerobic and anaerobic energy supplies (see page 34), which means they can be quite high-intensity activities.

Dance

Dance is not a very obvious choice of fitness activity, but you would be surprised at how enjoyable this cross-training activity is. You have a multitude of choice, too, and, though it might not give you quite the same aerobic workout as some of the other suggestions, it does have its own benefits. Try salsa, jive or belly dancing, or simply take an aerobic dance class at the gym. Other options include ballet, which is a beautiful skill to learn (yes, even as an adult!) and will improve your overall posture and give you great-looking legs.

If you can't find a class near you (try the Yellow Pages for dance classes and schools), there are a multitude of dance-inspired exercise videos on the market, which you can try out in the privacy of your own home.

04

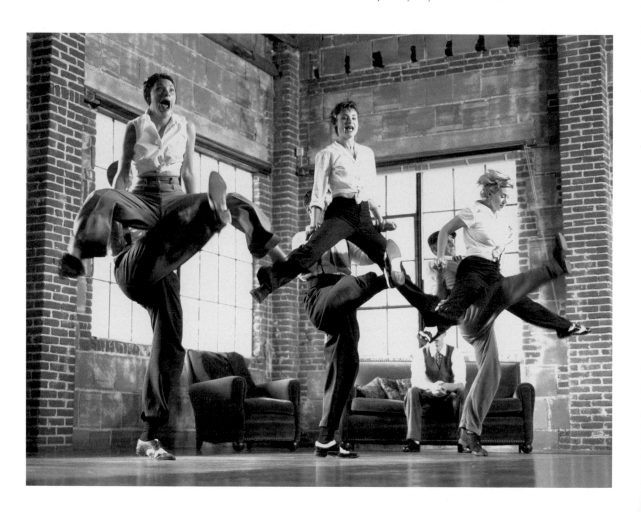

Building your combined workout

Week 1

Whatever your fitness level, start out by using the beginners' workout routine (see pages 76–85) for the first week. Set aside half an hour each time and try to practise this workout at least three times in the first week with a rest day between each session. There is no rush to master these skills, so don't try to run before you can walk.

Weeks 2–4

Aim to fit in two of the kick-boxing routines (pages 86–131), plus two troubleshooting workouts (pages 132–151). On top of this, add one session of your own cross-training activity. I suggest you pick one specific troubleshooting workout and concentrate on that. For example, if you wish to work on tightening your abdominal area, then just use that one for a few weeks. Make sure you have a rest day between each workout (see page 44). Your programme might look something like the one shown here.

Saturday	Cross-training workout
Sunday	REST
Monday	Kick-boxing workout plus abdominal routine
Tuesday	REST
Wednesday	REST
Thursday	Kick-boxing workout plus abdominal routine
Friday	REST

Weeks 4 onwards

After the initial few weeks you should be ready to move up a gear. Try following this routine, remembering to incorporate some rest days.

Saturday	REST
Sunday	Kick-boxing workout plus troubleshooting routine
Monday	REST
Tuesday	Cross-training workout (add troubleshooting routine if desired)
Wednesday	REST
Thursday	Cardio work only (such as speed walking, cycling or running)
Friday	Kick-boxing workout plus troubleshooting routine

Saturday	REST
Sunday	Kick-boxing workout plus troubleshooting routine
Monday	REST
Tuesday	Cardio workout only
Wednesday	Cross-training workout (add troubleshooting routine if desired)
Thursday	REST
Friday	Kick-boxing routine plus troubleshooting routine

THE WARM-UP AND COOL-DOWN

As with any form of exercise, the key to success in kick-boxing lies in the preparation. Without the warm-up exercises, you are failing to prepare yourself not only physically, but mentally too. During these exercises, the body is asked to adapt slowly (and therefore safely) to the increased blood and oxygen flow to the heart and muscles, while mentally you can work on focusing yourself on the workout to come.

The cool-down works on the same principle, but in reverse. The heart, although a strong and normally efficient muscle, needs adequate warning that its workload is about to decrease. Therefore, the cool-down allows the exercise intensity to reduce at a slow and steady pace.

You need to spend at least 5 minutes warming up before your body is ready for further work, and about the same amount of time cooling down at the end of your session. The main rule with the warm-up is to start slowly and build up gradually. With the cool-down, the key is not to suddenly stop exercising – decrease your level of activity slowly. A good analogy is to think of slowing down from a sprint to a fast run, through a jog and into a walk. All cool-downs and workouts should finish with a thorough stretch.

Please note that throughout this chapter and the workouts, I normally specify starting with a given leg or arm, and then changing over to the other side. There is no particular reason for starting with the right arm rather than the left, so do whichever feels more comfortable for you.

Why stretch?

Stretching is an important part of the process of cooling down and finishing off your workout. At this point your muscles are warm, so are ideally suited to enjoy the benefits of stretching (you should never stretch cold muscles). Your stretching programme should aim to increase mobility and enhance the elasticity of your muscles. It is important to look at stretching with a 'whole body' approach. There is no point being able to touch your toes if you can't do the zip up on the back of your dress!

The benefits of stretching

It increases the range of motion of each joint

Having a limited range of motion in certain joints may not be an issue for you while you are young (in fact you may not even be aware of it), but as you get older you may find problems developing. Not being able to cut your own toenails or reach up to the top shelf – it is these sorts of problems that can stem from a limited range of motion. So start stretching today!

It reduces muscle soreness after exercise

Delayed Onset Muscle Soreness (DOMS) is something you can experience in the 24–48-hour post-workout period. Scientific research suggests that this is due to tiny tears in muscle fibres caused by over-exertion. While stretching does not directly repair the tears in the fibres, it does help to maintain muscle elasticity, thereby reducing the risk of any future damage.

It reduces low-back pain

Anyone who has ever suffered from low-back pain knows how debilitating it can be. A lot of lower back problems are attributed to an imbalance in the muscles of the trunk and inappropriate flexibility in the pelvis. Stretching all the muscles will tend to sort out this imbalance.

It helps prevent injury

Risk of injuries, tissue tears and inflammation increases considerably if you suffer from poor flexibility. Therefore, a good stretching programme to improve your flexibility can minimize damage from all sorts of actions, from exercise and everyday activities to an unintentional fall.

It makes you feel good

Stretching is a great way to connect with your body. Use this time to focus on your body and how it feels as you stretch each part of it, and concentrate on feeling calm and relaxed.

WHAT ABOUT THE WARM-UP STRETCH?

There has been a lot of debate over the past few years on whether stretching before exercise (after your warm-up) is beneficial or whether it actually does more harm than good. The theory had always stood that the pre-workout stretch would not only reduce muscle soreness (by increasing muscle flexibility), but it could also reduce the chance of injury. However, various international studies have suggested that the decrease in the likelihood of injury is so small (about 5 per cent) that it is practically meaningless. That said, there are still many experts who believe there is a vital role for pre-exercise stretching. I suggest it comes down to common sense and individual choice. The most important thing to remember is that all experts agree that post-exercise stretching is imperative and should not be missed at all costs.

The warm-up

Make sure you begin every workout with a warm-up. Use the following exercises or, if you wish, spend 5–10 minutes either using home-exercise equipment (stationary bikes, rowers, etc.) or taking a brisk walk. Remember – start off slowly and build up the pace gradually.

05

Marching

Begin by marching on the spot, then move around the room if possible. Keep your feet softly flexed and don't slam them down. Keep your abdominal muscles tight and your back straight. Use your arms, keeping the elbows bent and the fists soft, pumping them backwards and forwards as you march.

Do: for 1 minute

Shoulder rolls

Keep marching with your feet and begin to roll your shoulders forwards. Let your arms hang loose by your sides and try to use the fullest range of motion possible. Work your shoulders forward, up, back then down.

Do: 5 rolls forwards, then reverse for 5 rolls.

Knee lifts

Lift alternate knees up in front of you, touching the lifted knee with the opposite hand. Don't lean forwards or backwards. Keep your back straight and abdominal muscles tight. Make sure your supporting knee remains soft (not locked).

Do: for 1 minute

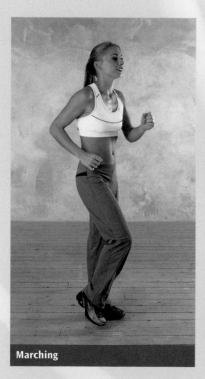
Marching

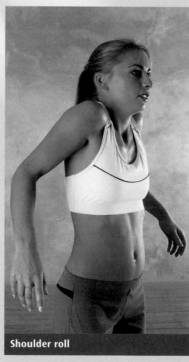
Shoulder roll

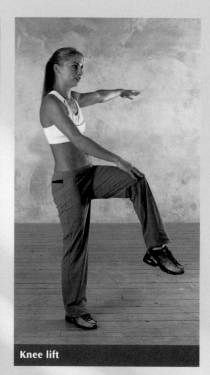
Knee lift

Neck rolls

Return to a march, keeping your back straight and your shoulders relaxed and down. Begin by taking your chin towards the right shoulder and slowly move your chin and head in a semi-circle down and over to the left shoulder, then reverse the process back to the right shoulder. Keep the movement slow and fluid.

Do: 8 times side to side

Heel digs

Stand with your feet hip-width apart and bring alternate heels forward, keeping the foot gently flexed. Your supporting knee should be soft and your back straight. Punch both arms out straight in front of you and then slowly raise your arms to increase the intensity of the exercise, until you are punching at 45° above head height.

Do: for 1 minute

Knee bends

Stand with your feet one-and-a-half times hip-width apart and your arms out in front of you. Keeping your back straight, flex at the knees and the hips. Make sure your knees travel in line with your toes and don't take your bottom any lower than the line of your knees. Straighten up, keeping your knees soft and not locking the joints.

Do: 8 times

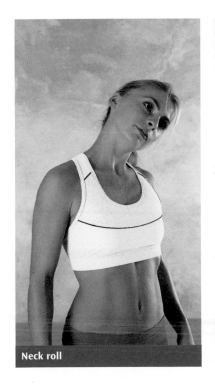

Neck roll

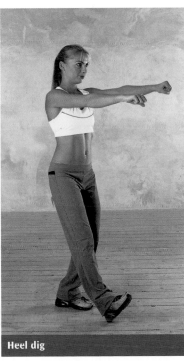

Heel dig

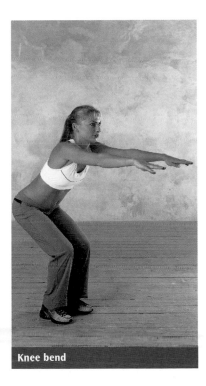

Knee bend

Pelvic circles

Stand with your feet hip-width apart, knees soft and back straight. Place your hands on your hips and gently circle your pelvis in a 'D' shape, straight across the back and around at the front. Try to isolate the movement to your hips, keeping your knees and upper body as still as possible.

Do: 5 times clockwise and 5 times anticlockwise

Side steps

Step side to side with long, easy strides. Place your feet down toes first, heels following. Keep your body upright and head lifted. Push your arms out in front of you at shoulder height with every stride.

Do: for 2 minutes

Leg curls

Add to the side steps by bringing alternate heels up towards your bottom. Make sure your supporting knee is soft and that you don't slam your feet down. Keep your arms at or above shoulder height, punching out with every leg curl.

Do: for 2 minutes

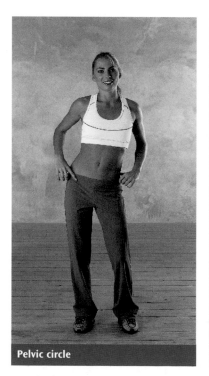

Pelvic circle

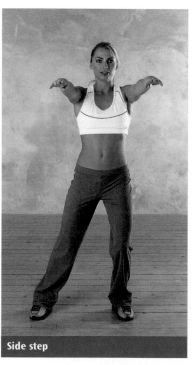

Side step

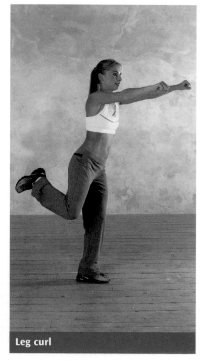

Leg curl

Warm-up stretches

If you decide you wish to include a short stretching component in your warm-up (see page 57), follow these stretches after the warm-up exercises (your muscles must be warm before stretching) and before the main workout.

Trapezius stretch

Stand with your feet hip-width apart and knees slightly bent. Link your hands, with your palms facing you, and reach out until you feel a stretch across the top of your back. Keep your elbows soft and your chin slightly down. Imagine you are hugging a beachball.

Back and side stretch

Stand with your feet one-and-half times hip-width apart and knees slightly bent. Place your right hand on your right hip and reach up and above your head with your left hand. Now lean over to your right, supporting your torso with the right hand. Aim to feel a stretch all along the left side. Change sides and repeat.

Chest and front-shoulders stretch

Clasp your hands together behind your back and lift them slightly away from the body. Keep your elbows bent, back straight and abdominals tight. Feel the stretch across the front of your chest.

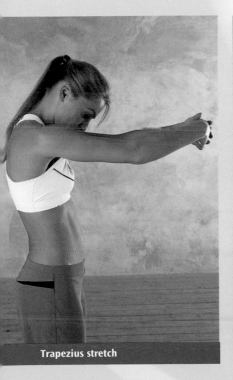

Trapezius stretch

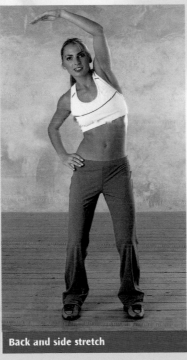

Back and side stretch

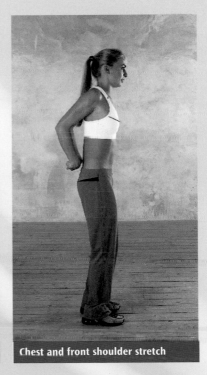

Chest and front shoulder stretch

Quad stretch

Use a wall for support if necessary. Keeping your back straight, flex your right knee and grasp the ankle behind you. Gently draw the heel to your bottom. Keep the supporting knee bent and try to keep your thighs parallel. Feel the stretch along the front of the bent thigh. Change legs.

Hamstring stretch

Bend your left knee and extend your right leg forwards, keeping the leg straight but not locking the knee. Place both hands on your left thigh and lean forwards over the bent leg, feeling the stretch along the back of the straight leg. Keep your back straight and abdominal muscles tight. Change legs.

Calf stretch

Start with your feet hip-width apart. Extend your right leg behind you while bending the left knee. Keep your hips and shoulders square and ensure your feet stay hip-width apart to maintain stability. Press your right heel into the floor and feel a stretch in the upper part of your right calf. Change legs.

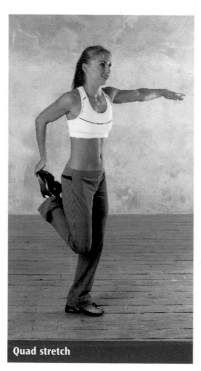

Quad stretch

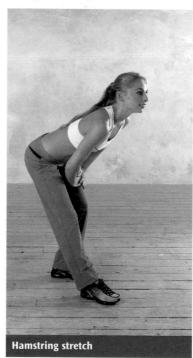

Hamstring stretch

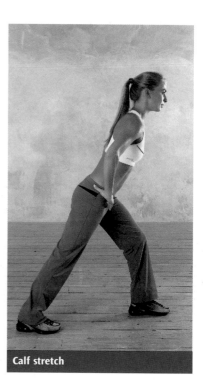

Calf stretch

STRETCHING TIPS
- Do each stretch once only and hold for about 10 seconds.
- Stretch to a point of tension, not pain.
- Keep breathing throughout.
- Don't bounce up and down while holding a stretch.

The cool-down

As with the warm-up, you can replace the routine shown below with other options, such as any home-exercise equipment or a brisk walk. Remember to start at a moderate pace and then decrease the intensity until you feel you have returned to your normal state. Always spend at least 5 minutes doing your cool-down and follow it with a stretching routine. Spend 30–60 seconds on each of the following:

Jog on the spot
Jog or march briskly on the spot.

Knee lifts with arms
Lift alternate knees up in front of you, touching each lifted knee with the opposite hand as you do so.

Knee lifts without arms
Continue the knee lifts, but with your hands on your hips.

Heel digs with bicep curls
Place alternate heels forwards on the floor in front of you. Hold your arms at your sides with the palms facing forwards in a loose fist. As you bring each foot forward, raise both hands to shoulder height, flexing at the elbow.

Heel digs without hands
Continue the heel digs, but with your hands on your hips.

Gentle marching on spot
Your pace should now slow right down as you finish off with gentle marching on the spot, before going on to your stretching routine.

REMEMBER TO:
- Spend 30–60 seconds on each exercise.
- Gradually reduce your pace throughout.
- Follow with a stretching routine.

Cool-down stretches

Calf stretch

Stand with your feet hip-width apart. Take your right leg back while bending the front knee, pressing the right heel into the ground. Keep your hips and shoulders square and ensure your feet stay hip-width apart for stability. Aim to feel this stretch in the upper part of the back calf. Hold for 20 seconds, then change legs.

Seated hamstring stretch

Sit with your left leg straight out in front of you and your right leg tucked comfortably in, with the foot against the opposite thigh. Sit up tall, then bend forwards from the hips over your straight leg. Try to keep the left foot gently flexed and the base of the knee relaxed into the ground. Come as far forward as feels comfortable for you, then hold the stretch. Try to keep your back as straight as possible. Hold for 20 seconds, then change sides.

Lying quad stretch

Lie on your front on the floor, with your head resting on your left hand. Bend your right leg and reach down with your right hand to grasp your right heel. Draw the heel towards your bottom. (If you have problems reaching your foot, wrap a towel or scarf around your ankle and use that to draw the foot up.) Keep your hips gently on the floor and your knees hip-width apart. Feel the stretch along the front of the bent thigh. Hold for 20 seconds, then change legs.

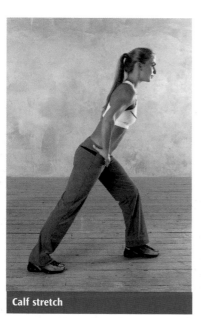

Calf stretch

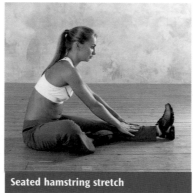

Seated hamstring stretch

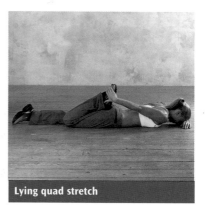

Lying quad stretch

HOW TO STRETCH

- Stretch gently – to the point of resistance not pain.
- Hold each stretch for about 20 seconds.
- Don't bounce up and down while holding a stretch. It can cause injury and muscle soreness.
- Keep breathing throughout.

Glute stretch

Lie with your back flat against the floor, your legs hip-width apart and the soles of your feet flat on the floor. Raise your right leg and cross it over the left leg, so it rests across your left thigh. Now raise your left leg so your left thigh is at almost 90° to the floor. At the same time, reach through and grasp your left thigh, gently drawing both legs towards you and feeling the stretch across your right buttock. Hold for 20–30 seconds, then release and change sides.

Lower-back ball

Lie on your back and draw your knees in towards your chest, hugging them with your arms. Make sure your head and neck are relaxed on the floor. Gently rock from side to side, massaging your spine into the floor. Continue for 20 seconds.

Hip-flexor stretch

Begin by kneeling up, then bring your right leg forwards into a right angle. Gently press your hips forwards, keeping your abdominal muscles tight and your body lifted, and taking care not to let your right knee go over the line of the toe. Feel the stretch in the front of your left hip and thigh. Hold for 20 seconds, then release and change sides.

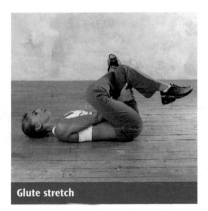

Glute stretch

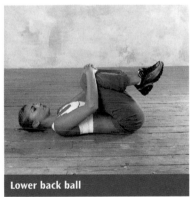

Lower back ball

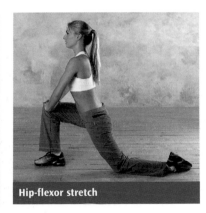

Hip-flexor stretch

- Keep warm – if necessary put on some extra layers of clothing before or during your stretches.
- If you have an injury, seek professional advice before stretching.
- Concentrate on the muscle you are stretching.
- Don't stretch cold muscles – make sure you have done an adequate warm-up and workout before starting any stretch programme.

Inner-thigh stretch

Sit on the floor and place the soles of your feet together, letting your knees drop open. Hold onto your ankles and gently try to press down on your thighs using your elbows. Keep your back straight and your spine tall and lifted. Hold for 20 seconds, then release.

Seated chest stretch

Sitting on the floor with your back straight, place both palms on the small of your back with the fingers pointing downwards. Squeeze your elbows towards each other, letting your chest open. Hold for about 20 seconds, then release.

Tricep stretch

Stretch your right arm up above your head, and drop your palm down between your shoulder blades. Now, with your left hand, gently press down on your right upper arm. Hold in this position for 20 seconds, then change sides.

05

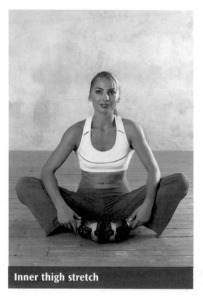

Inner thigh stretch

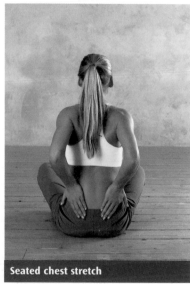

Seated chest stretch

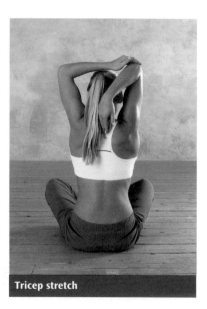

Tricep stretch

Tower stretch

Sitting with your back straight, interlock your fingers and, with your palms facing upwards, stretch your arms above your head. Make sure your elbows are straight and your upper arms pulled as far behind the ears as possible. Relax into the move and remember to breathe. Hold for about one minute before resting. Change the interlock of your fingers, so your other thumb is on top, then repeat.

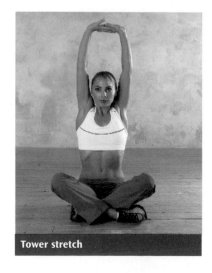

Tower stretch

Shoulder stretch

Swing your left arm across the front of your body and hook it in gently with your right forearm. Now gently draw the left arm across, feeling for a stretch in the back of the left shoulder. Hold for about 20 seconds, then change sides.

Back and side stretch

Kneeling up, place your right hand on your lower hip and stretch up tall with your left hand. Now stretch your left arm over your head, taking your body weight onto the right supporting hand. Hold for 20 seconds, then change sides.

Re-energizing jumps

This is the perfect way to finish off any stretching workout. Jump up and down a few times, keeping your knees and ankles soft. Think about being light on your feet – and smile!

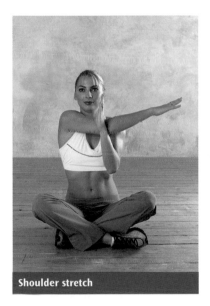

Shoulder stretch

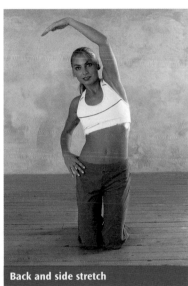

Back and side stretch

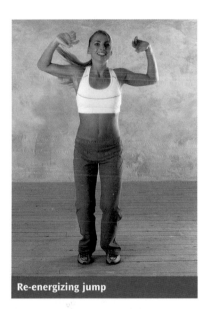

Re-energizing jump

Quick stretch routine

Please try to spend as much time as possible on your stretching routine. It is as important as the main workout. However, if you are in a rush, don't skimp on your technique or the time and care taken with each stretch. Just follow this shortened version of the above routine, adhering to the basic guidelines.

- Calf stretch (see page 64)
- Seated hamstring stretch (page 64)
- Lying quad stretch (page 64)
- Seated chest stretch (page 66)
- Back and side stretch (above)

KICK-BOXING BASICS

Before you get started on any of the workouts in this book, you need to spend some time working on the basic principles behind kick-boxing – namely, how to stand, move, kick and punch correctly. It is particularly important in kick-boxing that you don't rush ahead to the routines without having a good grasp of the techniques.

How to make a fist

Before you can punch anything, you need to know how to make a fist. It might sound simple enough but you would be amazed how many people get it wrong. What is also commonly misunderstood is that the fist is not clenched tight until it reaches the point of impact. Hands are held loose in readiness, even on the way to the target. Therefore, the fist tightens just before it lands and immediately relaxes as it is pulled back.

Don't wear rings or bracelets whilst training. If you have long fingernails, they may dig into your palms, so consider trimming them.

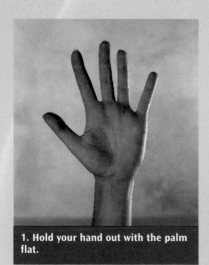

1. Hold your hand out with the palm flat.

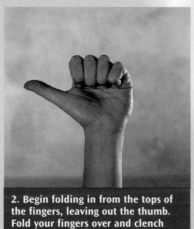

2. Begin folding in from the tops of the fingers, leaving out the thumb. Fold your fingers over and clench them into the palm.

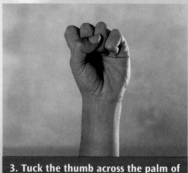

3. Tuck the thumb across the palm of the hand so it rests against the fingers. Your striking point is the two largest knuckles – that is, the knuckles where your index and third fingers join your hand.

Unless you have been studying kick-boxing or another martial art, it is unlikely you have kicked or punched anything (even thin air) for quite a while. Believe me, you are about to engage your muscles in a brand-new and very unfamiliar way. Not only is your body being asked to gain new skills quickly, but your brain is, too.

People spend years learning kick-boxing and honing their skills. Here, you are about to undertake a quick and simple course in the basics. Of course, you can learn a lot in a short time, but total mental and physical application is vital, so make sure you read, digest and practise the following principles before you get started on the routines.

The basic stance

Your first and most basic lesson is how to stand. Again, like making a fist, it might sound easy, but this is the foundation stone from which all your kicks and punches are thrown.

Your stance needs to be neutral – you don't want to be giving away your next move to your opponent, imaginary or otherwise. It also needs to balance your weight – 50 per cent on each leg – so you are in a position to throw any kicks or punches you desire. Your base of support and balance lies between your feet – you can't be pushed over if your feet are slightly more than shoulder-width apart.

To find your fighting stance, start with your feet hip-width apart. Step forwards a natural pace with your left foot, and angle your hips naturally with your feet. Let your back foot turn naturally so if points slightly outwards (on your clock, the back foot is at 5 o'clock). Make sure your knees are slightly bent. Though your body weight is distributed evenly between both feet, think about keeping this weight shifted towards the balls of your feet, rather than through the heels. Now for your arms: tuck your elbows in close to your sides, raising your forearms (as if you were holding daggers in your hands).

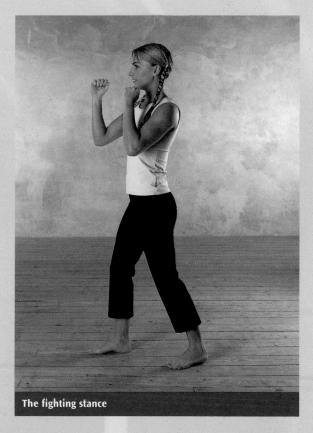

The fighting stance

How to punch safely

Left-handed or right?

A right-handed puncher fires 'power punches' with the right hand, standing with the left foot forward. Power punches are those like a cross or an uppercut that normally finish off a move. A short, sharp punch like a jab is done with the left hand to set up the power punch with the right.

However, if you are a natural left hander (called a 'southpaw' in boxing and kick-boxing), you will throw power punches with your left hand, with your right leg forward. Kick-boxers learn to throw kicks and punches from both sides, because kicks and punches can be fired from both sides.

06

Punches

• Your fist should be strong and tight, but don't grip too hard. Your hand shouldn't be so tense that you feel any strain in your forearm or wrist.

• Never fully extend your arm during a punch (you do not want to lock out the elbow joint).

• Always give yourself a mental target when you punch – think about punching about 30 cm (12 in) behind your target to make sure you punch 'through' it.

• Remember, a punch is not just thrown from the arms and shoulders, it requires correct whole-body mechanics behind it to make it safe and effective.

• Make sure you keep your fist, wrist and elbow in perfect alignment – they should be working in a flat plane throughout. Breathe out on every punch and inhale as you retract.

Punching dynamics

The great thing about punching is that it can give you an all-over workout – the power behind a punch begins in your toes. As you begin to throw the punch, the ball of your foot pivots; this then drives the legs through to the rotation of your hips. To help build the intensity of this power, your core muscles – those within the trunk of your body, including the abdominals and back muscles – also work. Then, as the punch is thrown, the entire arm, shoulder and chest muscles come into play. Finally, in

order to bring the punch quickly back, the big back muscles (latissimus dorsi, rhomboids and trapezius) have to do their bit. In short, everything has its part in throwing a successful punch.

Where do they land?

Even if you are only punching into thin air, it is important to know exactly where you are aiming for on your imaginary target. Punches are either to the head or to the body. On the head, aim for the chin or the lower jaw. When targeting the body, you should aim for the chest and stomach (you can cause most damage to your opponent by striking him or her in the upper part of the solar plexus, under the heart or in the liver area).

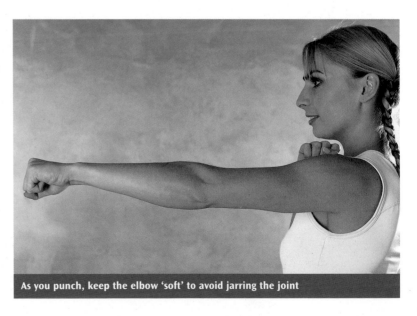

As you punch, keep the elbow 'soft' to avoid jarring the joint

How to kick safely

Kicks are your long-range weapons. Not only can you land a variety of kicks, you can also stop an opponent from getting too close. A powerful kick has more impact than a punch.

• Your mantra is 'chamber, execute, snap back, set down'. Say it again and again until it is ingrained.
• At no point should you lock your knee joints.
• Breathe out as you kick. Inhale as you retract.
• Keep your arms close to your body; resist the temptation to throw them out as you are learning to balance!

It is important to kick only where it feels comfortable for you. A high kick does not work muscles any more effectively than a low one. Concentrate on learning the kicks with proper technique at a low height while gradually increasing your flexibility. Then you can slowly build up height.

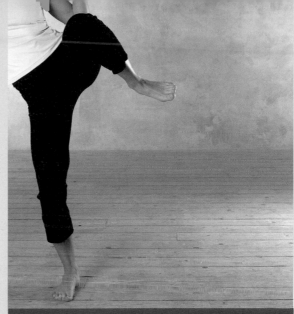

1. For effective kicking, always visualize your imaginary target, in the same way as you do with punching, and look towards it as you lift your kicking leg into what is called the chambered position.

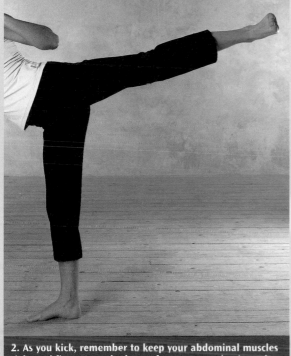

2. As you kick, remember to keep your abdominal muscles tight and firm. Keep the knee of your supporting leg soft and never fully extend your kicking leg.

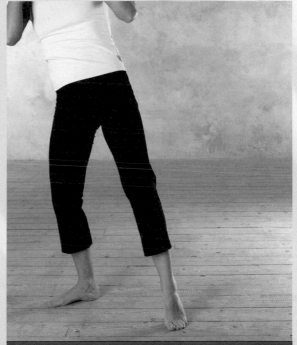

3. Don't slam the kicking foot down. Retract the kicking leg, following its original path, and place the foot down in its original position.

What muscles are you working?

Kicking mainly uses the muscles in your legs and bottom. Most kicks begin with the hip flexors (the area of muscle that picks up your knee). Then the muscle that runs down the front of your thigh (the quadriceps) helps execute the kick. The muscles at the back of your thigh (the hamstrings) and your bottom muscles themselves are all engaged, too, at one point. Finally, even your calf muscles (which you will use to support your entire body weight) get used, giving you an all-over lower-body workout.

Kicks and targets

As with punches, even if you are attacking an imaginary opponent, it is good to have some idea of the areas you are targeting. Have a look at the table opposite – the optimum column is the best place for you to land your kicks, while the secondary column lists targets which, in a sticky situation, could help you out!

Keeping moving

Now that you have a basic understanding of pivoting, kicking and punching, you will need to learn how to put them together. The first principle is how to move, or – in kick-boxing parlance – how to shuffle.

You can use shuffling to get close to your opponent as well as away from him or her. It is nothing more than a step–drag. Move forwards by stepping with the lead foot first, dragging the rear. Move back by stepping with the rear foot first, dragging the front. Move to either side by stepping first with the foot on that side, dragging the second foot. Close the gap between your feet quickly. The idea is that you maintain the integrity of your fighting stance, not overstepping, crossing over or bringing the feet together. Spend time practising, applying this technique first to punches and then to kicks. Try travelling the length of a room or open space, then turning around and using the opposite leg to go back.

Striking surfaces

The next thing you need to know is what you should be kicking with! If you kick an opponent or bag with the wrong part of your foot, you can really hurt yourself (see photos, right).

A bit about blocks

In this book you will learn to kick-box as a means to an end – to help lose excess body fat. In real-life training, the kicks, punches and stances that you are taught here are only the tip of the iceberg. You would also be learning a lot about defending yourself (blocking other people's attacks) and about sparring (fighting). Everybody needs to learn how to act defensively (blocks) as well as offensively (kicks and punches) before they can begin to have a comprehensive knowledge of any martial art. So please do not think that this book is going to equip you for any real-life fighting situations. If you want to learn kick-boxing in a more in-depth manner, please refer to our list of recommended teachers, clubs and associations which can be found at the back of the book (see page 157).

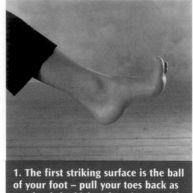

1. The first striking surface is the ball of your foot – pull your toes back as you land the kick, otherwise you risk smashing them.

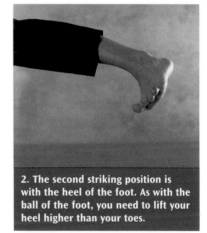

2. The second striking position is with the heel of the foot. As with the ball of the foot, you need to lift your heel higher than your toes.

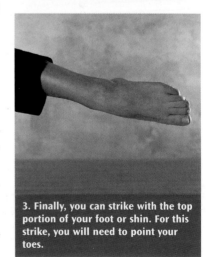

3. Finally, you can strike with the top portion of your foot or shin. For this strike, you will need to point your toes.

Pivoting

When kicking, your supporting leg is very important. Not only is the supporting ankle taking all your body weight during your kicks, but it is also maintaining your balance. Therefore, how you pivot the rest of your body on this foot is integral to your whole body movement. To gain full momentum and power in kicking, your ankle must work in unison with your knees and hips. If you pivot through the top half of your body, leaving the standing knee and ankle behind, many an injury can occur.

First, you need to make sure your feet begin in the correct position for the particular stance, punch or kick. Keep your body weight off the heel and focused towards the ball of the foot. Be aware of which way your foot (and therefore body) is going to be moving. Remember the foot is the start point of the pivot – everything else is going to follow through simultaneously. Always look in the direction you are turning.

Spend time practising pivoting. You can do this by practising standing and balancing on one leg. For example: begin in fighting stance with the left leg behind, now lift up the front right leg into your 'chambered' position, pivoting through on the left ankle. Hold for a count of five and then set the front foot down and repeat.

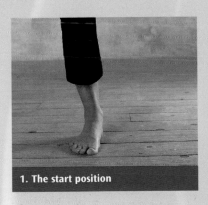

1. The start position

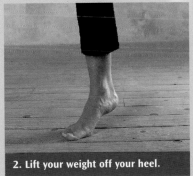

2. Lift your weight off your heel.

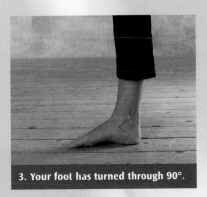

3. Your foot has turned through 90°.

Kicks	Optimum target area	Secondary target area
Front kick	stomach, groin, thigh	chest
Side kick	stomach	chest, groin
Round kick	side head, kidney, thigh	stomach
Roundhouse	side head, kidney, groin	chest, stomach
Straight knee	stomach, groin	side head
Side knee	kidney, stomach	side head

THE WORKOUTS

A good kick-boxer can be as graceful as a ballet dancer – it is all in the movement. Just think of the phrase associated with Muhammad Ali – 'float like a butterfly, sting like a bee' – and you will have the right idea. Of course, this type of grace takes time and practice to acquire, but it is well worth the effort.

Think about being light on your feet at all times and get used to being on the balls of your feet. If you lean back on your heels, you will lose your natural balance. Practise shadow boxing in front of a mirror and spend time putting all the different techniques you learn within the workouts together (in fact, it is a great idea to do the entire workout in front of a mirror, if possible). Blend combinations of kicks and punches and try to find your own flow and rhythm. At first, you may feel silly and rather vain, dancing around in front of a mirror, but it really is the best way for you to see any faults and imperfections in your technique, and so for you to improve.

The following workouts are spilt into three levels: beginners', intermediate and advanced. The beginners' workout will teach you the basic kicks and punches, plus some simple combinations. Just because you master the basics doesn't mean you never have to do the beginners' routine again. In fact, it is advisable to go back to it once in a while to help refine your technique in the basic kicks and punches. It can also be used as an extra warm-up routine when you move on to the intermediate and advanced levels. Whatever routine you choose to work on, ensure you always warm up first, then cool down and stretch after your workout.

Interspersed with these workouts are three routines that have been generously contributed to this book by other kick-boxing teachers and martial-arts practitioners. Natasha Redfern, Martin Ace, Kerry-Louise Norbury and Cris Janson-Piers are all experts in their field, and you can use

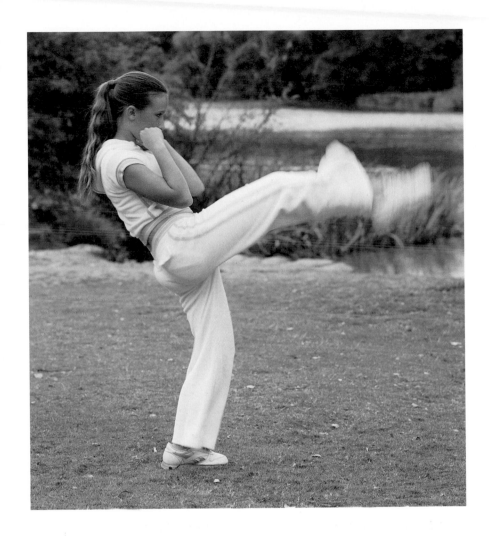

their suggestions as a change from mine. Please note that Kerry and Cris's workout is very advanced and shouldn't be tried at home – it's here to show you what you can aspire to if you really decide to take kick-boxing seriously.

A note on timing, whether you are using my workouts or anyone else's. As I said at the start of Chapter Five, you should spend at least 5 minutes at the start of your exercise session stretching and warming up, and at least a further 5 minutes at the end cooling down. In between, you should spend about 20–30 minutes on the workout itself. Do this three times a week and you will be amazed at the difference it makes to your fitness and overall well-being.

BEGINNERS' WORKOUT

Make sure you do a warm-up before you get started (see pages 58–62). Aim to work at 70 per cent of your maximum heart rate (see page 41, for information on calculating your MHR and measuring your heart rate). This workout is suitable for all levels of experience, although you should have a grasp of the basics as shown in Chapter Six (see pages 68–73). It involves some basic punches and kicks (including the jab, cross, hook, front kick, roundhouse kick and side kick) which form the building blocks of kick-boxing.

Exercise 1 – combination

Jab

1 Start in the fighting stance with your right leg behind. Make sure your weight is evenly distributed between both legs. Keep your knees slightly bent and your back heel slightly off the floor. Keep your arms up with your fists gently closed.

2 To jab, snap your leading (left) fist out towards the target, taking care not to fully extend the arm (locking the elbow). As the hand leaves its guard position next to your chin, the fist rotates through 90 degrees. The jab snaps out, with the fist clenching just before reaching the target, and is pulled back immediately. A quick recovery is as important as a quick delivery.

Cross

1 Begin in fighting stance.

2 This punch is made with your back hand. It begins with a hip twist, which drives the punching hand forwards and the back heel off the floor. Make sure you use your shoulders, waist and hips to help deliver the punch. Your front leg should be slightly bent, and your weight should shift forwards as you complete the punch. Don't lock the punching elbow. Retract the punch quickly back to your original stance.

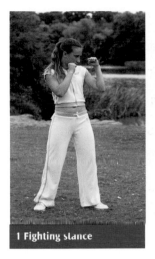
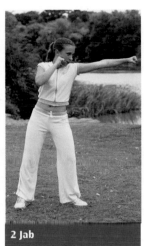
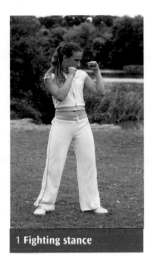
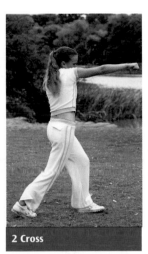

1 Fighting stance

2 Jab

1 Fighting stance

2 Cross

Jab–cross

1 Start in fighting stance.

2 Your front-arm jab is a small, quick movement.

3 Follow this immediately with a cross from your back hand, then return to the fighting stance.

Do

Right leg behind – 10 jabs with left arm, 10 crosses with right arm, 10 jab–cross combinations
Change legs
Left leg behind – 10 jabs with right arm, 10 crosses with left arm, 10 jab–cross combinations

Cardio break – skipping

You can skip with or without a rope. However, using a rope is much more effective and a great way to burn excess calories. Skip with both feet together or with one foot leading, but don't try to jump too high. Keep your knees and ankles soft at all times. If you are a novice to skipping, you'll be amazed how long just 20–30 seconds feels, so begin slowly and build up. Increase the length of time of your cardio break to 2–3 minutes if you are an experienced skipper or you wish to make the workout more intense.

Do

30–60 seconds

Exercise 2

Hook

1 The hook is a compact power punch. Begin in fighting stance with your right leg behind. You are going to 'throw a hook' off your front left hand. The punch begins with a weight transfer to your left side. From fighting stance the left elbow is bought up, almost parallel to the floor, so that the arm forms a sort of hook (hence the name). At the same time, the fist is rotated either palm down for a very close target or palm-in for targets further away.

2 The punch is delivered by pivoting the left foot, left leg and torso sharply to the right in a powerful, single torquing action (the arm does not move independently). Allow the hook to accelerate towards the target, the fist clenching before impact, and return it sharply to the fighting position.

Do

Right leg behind – 20 left hooks
Change legs
Left leg behind – 20 right hooks

Cardio break – skipping

Do

30–60 seconds

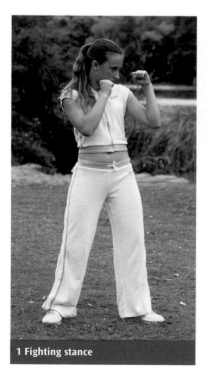

1 Fighting stance

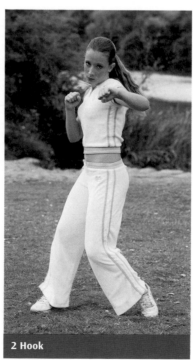

2 Hook

Exercise 3

Front kick

1 To perform a front kick, stand in fighting stance with your right leg behind.

2 From here, turn your hips to the front, raising your right knee to your chest (this is called 'chambering' the kick).

3 Now extend the kick towards the target, delivering the kick with the ball of the foot. The upper body moves slightly back, letting the hips move forward. As you kick, let this forward thrust of the hips generate the power behind the kick. Snap the lower leg back quickly to the chambering position and set it down in your original fighting stance.

Do
Right leg behind – 15 kicks with right leg
Change legs
Left leg behind – 15 kicks with left leg

Cardio break – skipping

Do
30–60 seconds

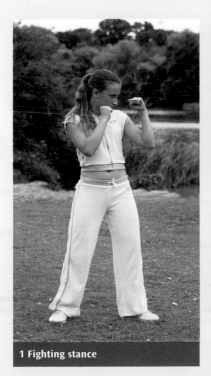

1 Fighting stance

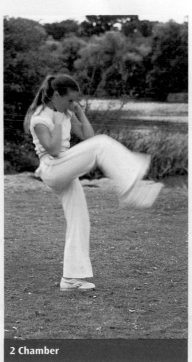

2 Chamber

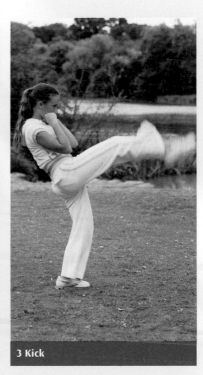

3 Kick

Exercise 4

Roundhouse kick

1 Start in fighting stance with your right leg behind.

2 Lift your right leg up into its chambered position by squaring the hips to the front. As you do this, turn the toes so they point downwards.

3 Begin the kick by pivoting the hips towards the left and extend the kick to its target, making contact with the top of your foot. Bring the kick back to its chambered position, spinning round on your supporting leg and turning the hips to the right (so they are square again). Place the foot down quickly in its original position. The kick's power comes from the snapping motion and the torque of the hips turning as the kick is delivered.

Do

Right leg behind – 15 kicks with right leg
Change legs
Left leg behind – 15 kicks with left leg

Cardio break – skipping

Do

30–60 seconds

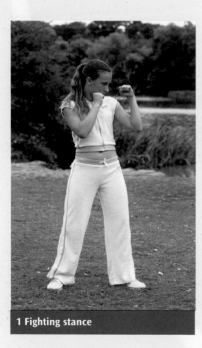

1 Fighting stance

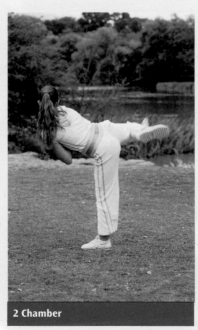

2 Chamber

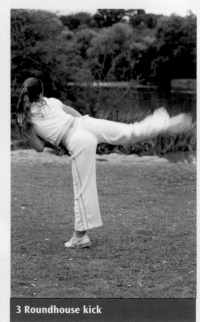

3 Roundhouse kick

Exercise 5

Side kick

1 Begin in fighting stance with your left leg behind. This kick is going to be delivered with the base of your left heel.

2 Raise your left leg into its chambered position by turning the hips square towards the front. As you chamber the kick, drop your toes so that they are pointing downwards. Rotate the hips almost 90° to the left, keeping the kicking leg in chamber.

3 As the leg snaps out into the kick, allow your hips to roll over towards your target – this is called 'turning into the kick'. Even though your body is turned slightly away from the opponent, don't take your eyes off the target. The kick thrusts out in a straight line. Make sure the heel is slightly higher than the toes to help land the kick. Snap the kicking leg back into chamber with the hips still in a side position. Set the foot down quickly in your original fighting stance.

Do
Left leg behind – 15 kicks with left leg
Change legs
Right leg behind – 15 kicks with right leg

Cardio break – skipping

Do
30–60 seconds

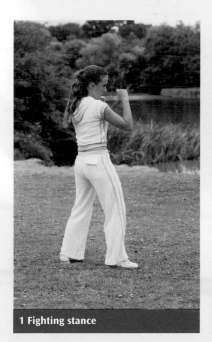
1 Fighting stance

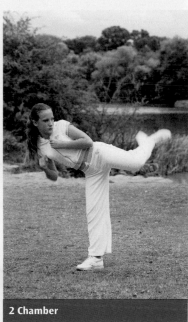
2 Chamber

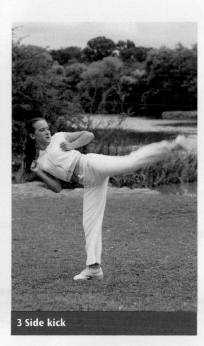
3 Side kick

Exercise 6 – combination

Jab–roundhouse

1 Begin in fighting stance with your right leg behind.

2 Throw a jab with the lead (left) hand.

3 As the jab recoils, bring the rear shoulder and leg forward to launch a roundhouse. Place the kicking leg back down in the original fighting stance.

Do
Right leg behind – 10 jab–roundhouse combinations
Change legs
Left leg behind – 10 jab–roundhouse combinations

Cardio break – skipping

Do
30–60 seconds

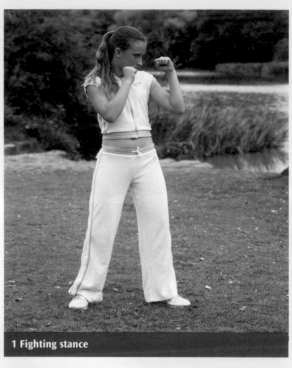

1 Fighting stance

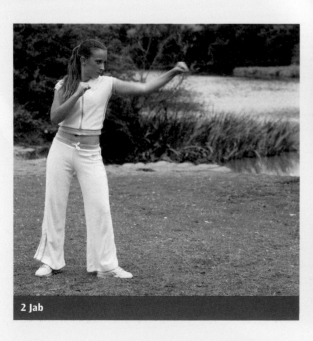

2 Jab

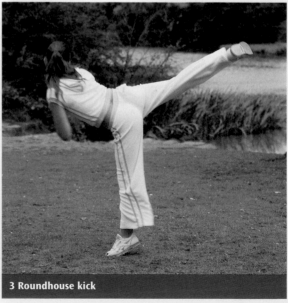

3 Roundhouse kick

Exercise 7 – combination

Front kick–jab–cross

1 Begin in fighting stance with your right leg behind.

2 Throw a front kick off your rear (right) leg.

3 Set the kicking leg down and fire a jab with your left hand.

4 Follow with a cross from the right. Return to fighting stance.

Do
Right leg behind – 10 front-kick–jab–cross combinations
Change legs
Left leg behind – 10 front-kick–jab–cross combinations

Cardio break – skipping

Do
30–60 seconds

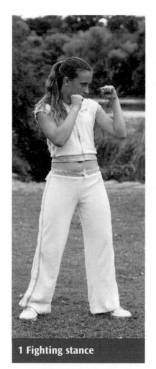
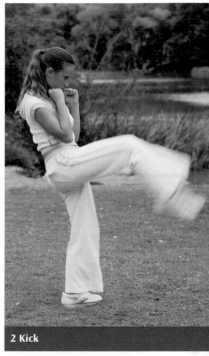

1 Fighting stance **2 Kick**

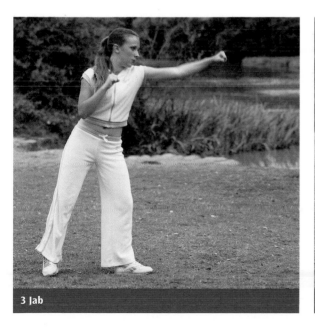
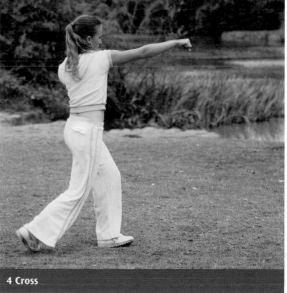

3 Jab **4 Cross**

Exercise 8

Uppercut

1 Uppercuts are thrown with power coming up from the legs and torso. Begin in fighting stance with your right leg behind. Dip the left shoulder so your elbow nears your hip. At the same time, rotate the fist palm up. Without cocking the arm back, propel this punch with the left side of your body. Accelerate, hit target and recover.

2 An uppercut from your rear hand can be thrown in the same way.

Do

Right leg behind – 10 uppercuts with left arm, 10 uppercuts with right arn, 10 uppercuts with left then right arms
Change legs, then with left leg behind – 10 uppercuts with right arm, 10 uppercuts with left arm, 10 uppercuts with right then left arms

Cardio break – skipping

Do
30–60 seconds

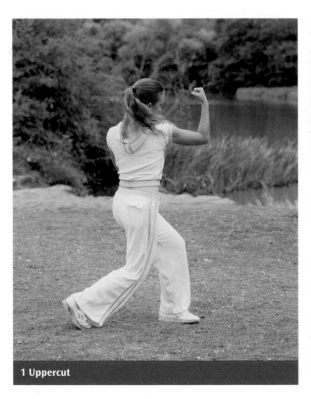

1 Uppercut

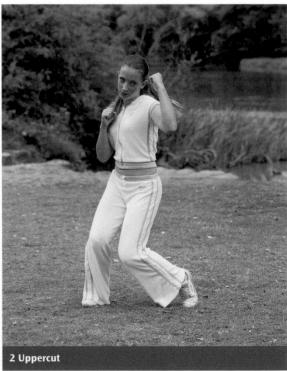

2 Uppercut

Exercise 9

Front and rear elbow

1 Start in fighting stance with your right leg behind. Raise the front left elbow into a horizontal position, with your hand close to your shoulders. Do not make a tight fist though, because a closed fist will tighten the forearm muscles and make the strike slower. Snap the left shoulder forward with the left elbow leading. As the elbow hits the target, retract the arm back to the original position.

2 To throw a rear elbow strike (one with the back arm), start in fighting stance, with your right leg behind. Twist the upper body forward with the right shoulder leading the way. As the right shoulder is coming forward, raise the right arm into the horizontal position. The right hand will be close to the right shoulder. As the arm snaps forward, the elbow

extends out and hits the target. After it lands on the target, snap the elbow back.

Do

Right leg behind – 10 elbows with left arm, 10 elbows with right arm, 10 elbows with left then right arms
Change legs
Left leg behind – 10 elbows with right arm, 10 elbows with left arm, 10 elbows with right then left arms

Cool-down and stretch

Finish your workout with the cool-down routine and a long stretch (see pages 63–67).

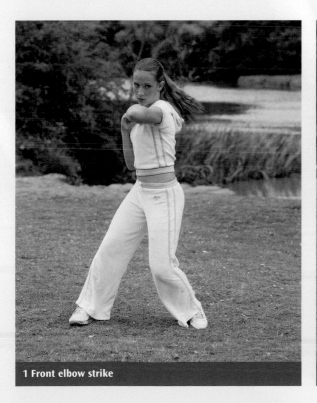
1 Front elbow strike

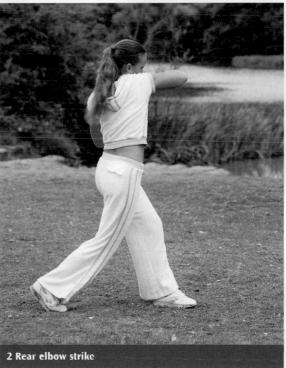
2 Rear elbow strike

BOX-A-CISE CLASS

NATASHA REDFERN

Natasha (like so many others) found her career path in health and fitness without really trying. After finishing school, she spent a year at university studying art, but it was during this period that she realized this wasn't what she was happiest doing. She decided to try her hand first at massage, then at aerobics. From this point on, Natasha was off and running – by increasing her qualifications and knowledge base in the health-and-fitness industry, she became the sought-after personal-fitness trainer she is today.

Though naturally twig-like (her own words), Natasha first changed her own physique to a more athletic and healthy size and then moved on to being very successful in changing other people's (usually the fuller figure) to their optimum weights. Her top tips for successful fat loss are:

• First and foremost, make sure you choose a form of exercise you enjoy.

• Fit in 30-minute sessions of aerobic work three times a week – without fail. Once a week is OK for maintenance of weight and fitness level, twice a week will produce a little development in your fitness, but three times is essential if you really want to see results.

• Always try to incorporate some weight training into your fitness programme to help increase lean muscle and boost your metabolism.

• Remember, you have to put the work in yourself! Don't expect great results from minimum effort. However, if you work hard you will always see results.

The workout

Try following this one of Natasha's very successful boxing-inspired fat-burning workouts. An understanding of the basics given in the beginners' workout (see pages 76–85) will be sufficient to tackle these moves. She recommends putting on some music (quite a fast beat – about 136–145 beats per minute) and keeping up with the rhythm as you work. Remember, the more intensity and power you put into this routine the more you will get out of it. However, if you are a beginner to exercising to music then always start slowly and build up gradually. Use our basic warm-up routine to start this aerobic workout. Run through exercises 1–7 twice, then finish with a cool-down and stretch. Aim to be working at 70–75 per cent of your MHR (see page 41), depending on your level of fitness.

Left jab–right cross

Throw a combination of first a left jab, then a right cross.

Do
1–2 minutes

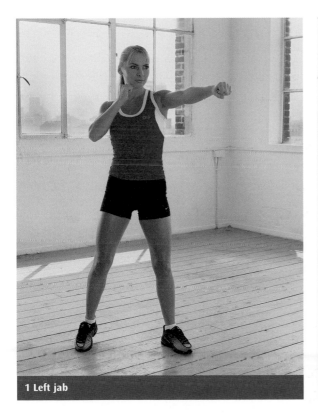

1 Left jab

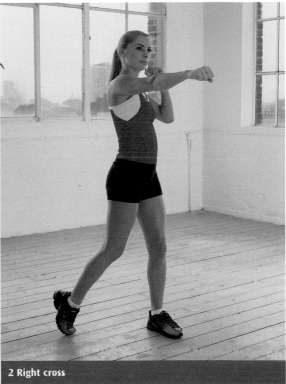

2 Right cross

Left hook–right hook

Throw a combination of a left hook followed by a right hook.

Do

1–2 minutes

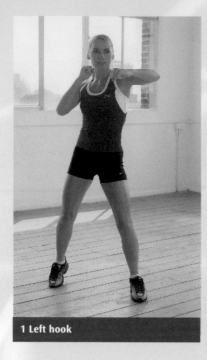

1 Left hook

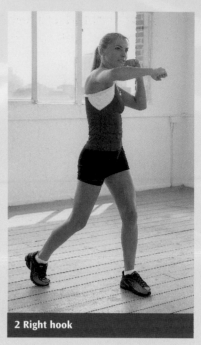

2 Right hook

Right uppercut–left uppercut

Throw a combination of a right uppercut followed immediately by a left one.

Do

1–2 minutes

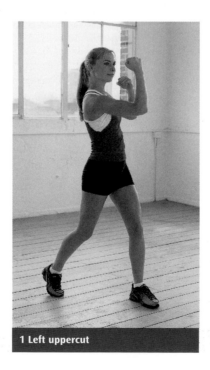

1 Left uppercut

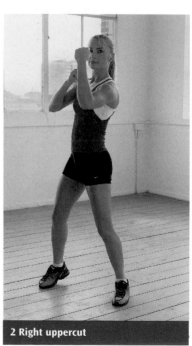

2 Right uppercut

Left hook–right uppercut

Start with a left hook following through with a right uppercut.

Do
1–2 minutes

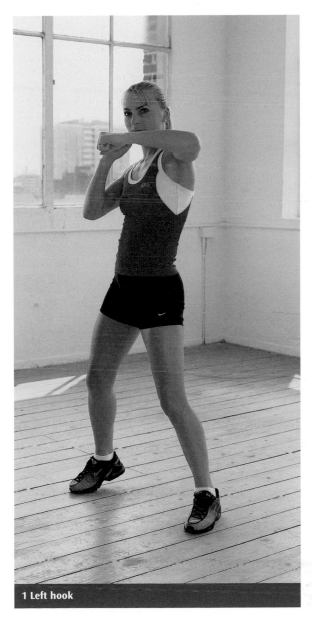

1 Left hook

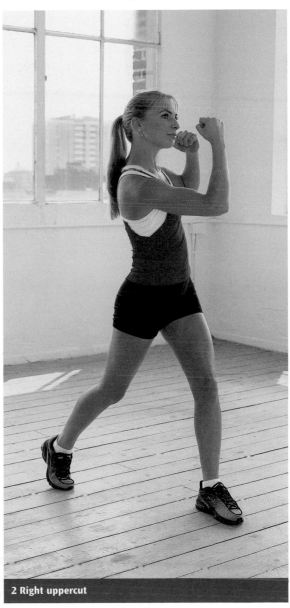

2 Right uppercut

Right hook–left uppercut

Begin with a right hook, following through with a left uppercut.

Do

1–2 minutes

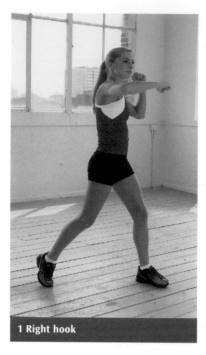

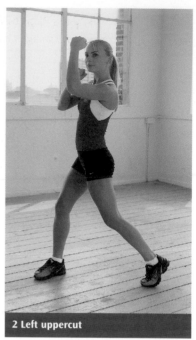

1 Right hook

2 Left uppercut

Left jab–left uppercut

Begin with a left jab, then a left uppercut.

Do

1–2 minutes

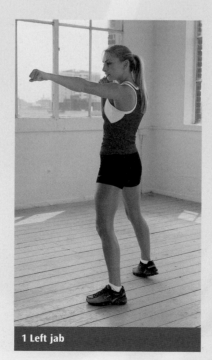

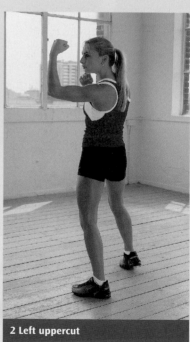

1 Left jab

2 Left uppercut

Right jab – right uppercut

Throw a right jab, following through with a right uppercut

Do

1–2 minutes

Cool-down and stretch

When you have run through exercises 1–7 twice, finish off with a cool-down and stretching routine (see pages 63–7).

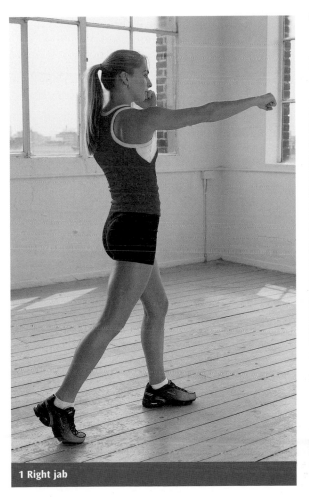

1 Right jab

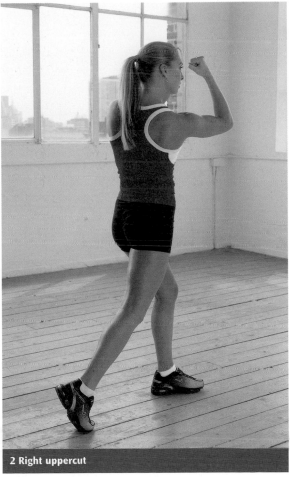

2 Right uppercut

INTERMEDIATE WORKOUT

This workout is designed for you to move on to when you feel completely confident with all the basic moves you have learned in the beginners' workout. Now you are being asked to perform slightly more complicated combinations and to learn a few more advanced moves.

Mentally, you are being asked to be a little more on the offensive. To help you mentally build an offensive mode, begin to create your imaginary opponent, so your new combinations become ways of attacking this invisible foe. Your kicks are now being thrown high or low, and you need to be light on your feet. Imagine this opponent attacking you from all sides with a variety of moves – you need to be on your toes and on the ball to keep the upper hand.

Remember you can always use the beginners' workout as a quick refresher course in the basic techniques – it doesn't mean you are going backwards in your fitness goals. All good martial artists (and athletes of any description) regularly return to basics in order to improve their skills further.

The intermediate workout is divided into two levels. Start off with level one for your first few sessions, progressing to level two when you feel ready.

To begin, follow the warm-up (see pages 58–62), then use exercises 1 and 3 of the beginners' workout (jab–cross combination and front kick, see pages 76–7 and 79) to prepare yourself further. Start by throwing these kicks and punches at a medium pace with minimum power and build up slowly, then continue immediately into the intermediate workout, following level one or two, depending on your individual fitness level. Aim to be working at 75–80 per cent of your MHR (see page 41).

Exercise 1 – combination

Jab–cross–hook–uppercut

1 Begin in fighting stance with your right leg behind.

2 Throw a jab off your front left hand. Let it snap towards its target and pull back quickly.

3 Follow this immediately with a right cross. Remember to use your hips and let the back heel come off the floor.

4 Now throw a hook with your front left hand, pivoting your left foot, left leg and torso sharply to the right.

5 Finish off the combination with a right-hand uppercut.

Do

Level one:
right leg behind – 20 combinations
left leg behind – 20 combinations

Level two:
right leg behind – 30 combinations
left leg behind – 30 combinations

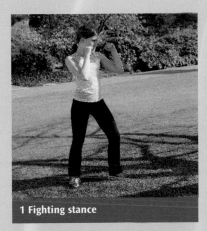

1 Fighting stance

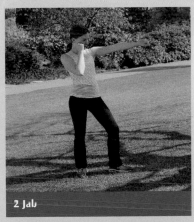

2 Jab

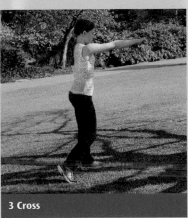

3 Cross

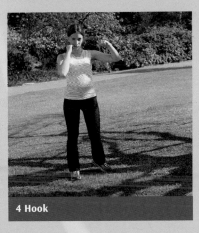

4 Hook

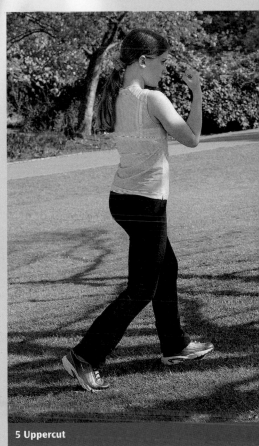

5 Uppercut

Exercise 2 – combination

Jab–spinning back fist

1 Begin in fighting stance with your right leg behind.

2 Throw a jab with your lead (left) hand.

3 Then perform a spin throw by turning clockwise on your front foot, leading with your right shoulder. As your body spins round to face the front again, whip your right arm out in a horizontal position. Your fist should be vertical. Imagine you are striking your target with the back part of your hand. After the strike, you will finish with the opposite foot forward. Return your right arm back into your normal fighting stance, now with the left leg behind.

To repeat, throw the next jab with the right hand and follow throw with another spinning back fist, but now with the left arm.

Do
Level one:
right leg behind – 20 combinations
left leg behind – 20 combinations

Level two:
right leg behind – 30 combinations
left leg behind – 30 combinations

Cardio break – skipping

Do
1–2 minutes

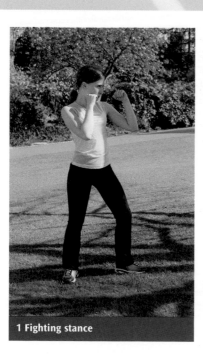

1 Fighting stance

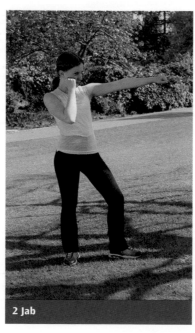

2 Jab

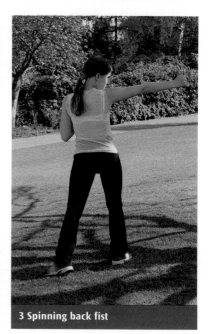

3 Spinning back fist

Exercise 3 – combination

Low roundhouse–high round kick

1 Begin in fighting stance with your left leg behind.

2 Throw a low left-leg roundhouse, aimed to strike your opponent's thigh. Don't re-chamber the kick; instead, drop the kicking leg in front (so you are now in your fighting stance with the right leg behind).

3 Follow through with a high left-leg round kick to your opponent's head. First, remember the kick's power comes from the snapping motion and the torque of the hips as it is delivered. Secondly, do not push yourself past your body's natural limits – if you cannot reach your second kick to head height, then aim for the torso instead. The ability to kick high comes with practice and doesn't necessarily mean you need extra power and strength.

Do

Level one:
right leg behind – 15 combinations
left leg behind – 15 combinations

Level two:
right leg behind – 25 combinations
left leg behind – 25 combinations

Cardio break – skipping

Do
1–2 minutes

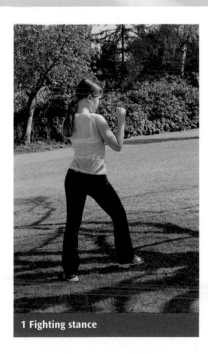

1 Fighting stance

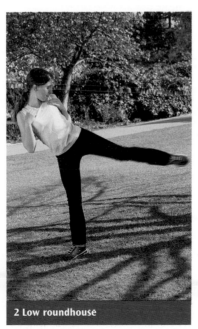

2 Low roundhouse

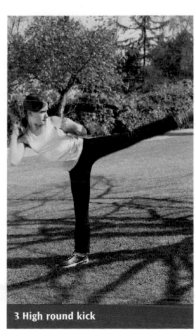

3 High round kick

Exercise 4 – aerobic kicks

Practising aerobic kicks is a way to work on the speed and technique of a particular kick. Aim for precise technique first, then build up the speed – you should be getting out of breath and working up a sweat. Start learning this particular kick by practising leg swings. This will help you limber up the muscles involved and, eventually, build up the height and speed of the kick itself.

Stand in fighting stance with your right leg behind. Your hands can either be in the fighting-stance position or hanging loosely by your sides. Start by swinging the right leg up to roughly waist height. Keep the right foot gently flexed and don't lock the knee. The supporting leg should be soft, too. Return to the start position and repeat immediately. This should be a flowing, swinging exercise with the emphasis on loosening up the hamstrings (the muscles running down the back of your thigh) and building up the height of the swing itself. Aim to take the leg slightly higher each time. Do 20–25 swings on the right leg, then change sides. When you feel adequately limbered up, try the axe kick itself.

Axe kicks

The axe kick's weapon is the heel; it is primarily used to attack the head, shoulders and chest. The leg's high chopping motion gives the kick its name. The kick itself needs to be set up in combination with other kicks and punches to be truly effective – however you are going to learn and use it as a single kick for the purposes of this workout.

1 Start in fighting stance with your right leg behind. Begin the kick by raising the right leg, keeping the knee slightly bent. As you raise your leg, turn your hips towards the left. Raise the leg in an arc-like shape, angling to the point directly above the target. As you chop down onto the target, twist

your hips to the right. Drop the leg down through the target and replace it in the original fighting stance.

Do
Level one:
right leg behind – 20 kicks
left leg behind – 20 kicks

Level two:
right leg behind – 30 kicks
left leg behind – 30 kicks

Cardio break – skipping

Do
1–2 minutes

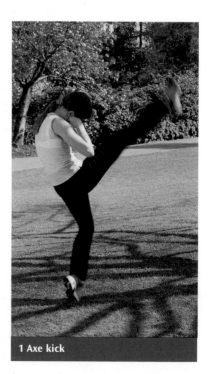

1 Axe kick

Exercise 5 – combination

Knee strikes are very powerful weapons and, regardless of your size, very effective. You can strike to a number of targets: legs, groin, stomach or head. By holding onto your opponent's head, you generate more power. The most common type of grab is a double-handed grip, bringing your elbows together to make a vice-like hold around the neck.

By grabbing the neck, you can throw off your opponent's balance and stabilize your own. As with all the kicks and punches in this book, these are not things to be taken lightly so do not try practising on real people without professional supervision.

Jab–cross–rear knee strike

1 Begin in fighting stance with your right leg behind. Throw a jab with the front left hand.

2 Follow through the jab with a right cross.

3 Now grab your imaginary opponent and fire a rear knee strike. Do this by grabbing the neck of your imaginary opponent, then shift your weight to your front leg and pull the neck of your opponent down. At the same time, shoot your rear knee straight up and deliver the strike to your opponent's head with the bone just above your kneecap. Return the leg back to your original fighting stance.

Do
Level one:
right leg behind – 20 combinations
left leg behind – 20 combinations

Level two:
right leg behind – 30 combinations
left leg behind – 30 combinations

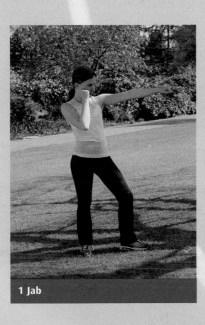

1 Jab

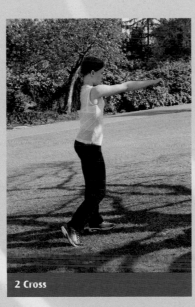

2 Cross

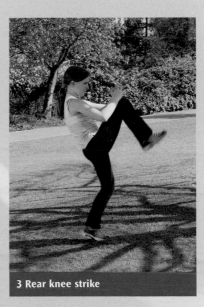

3 Rear knee strike

Exercise 6 – aerobic kicks

This part of the workout is designed to make you hot, out of breath and sweaty! Make these kicks precise, with good technique and as fast as you can.

Side kicks

1 Begin in fighting stance with your left leg behind.

2 Perform the side kicks with the rear left leg, remembering to let the leg snap and the hips roll over into the kick. Make sure the kick thrusts out in a straight line. Keep the supporting knee slightly bent and ensure you pivot correctly through the supporting ankle.

Do
Level one:
right leg behind – 20 kicks
left leg behind – 20 kicks

Level two:
right leg behind – 30 kicks
left leg behind – 30 kicks

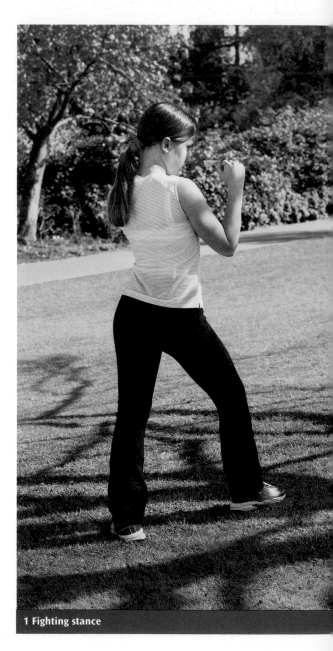

1 Fighting stance

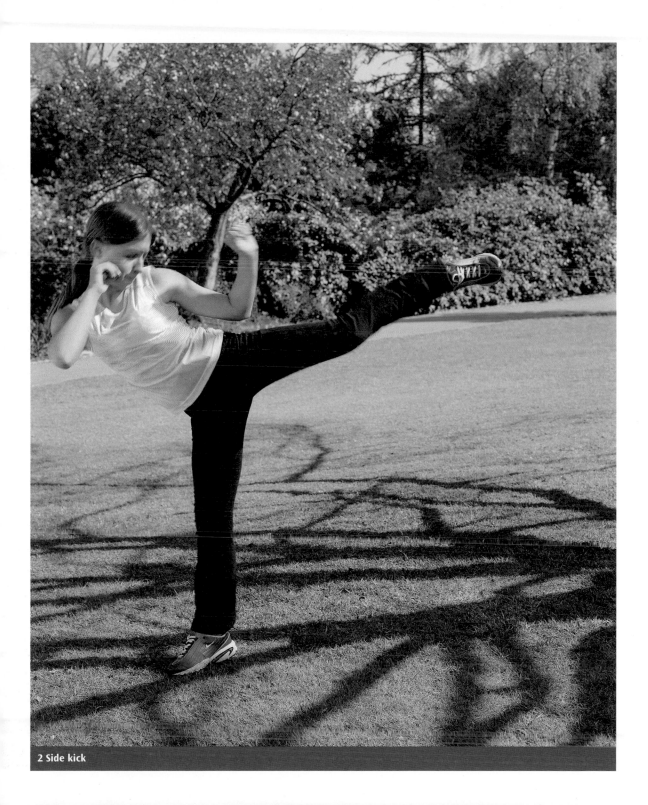

2 Side kick

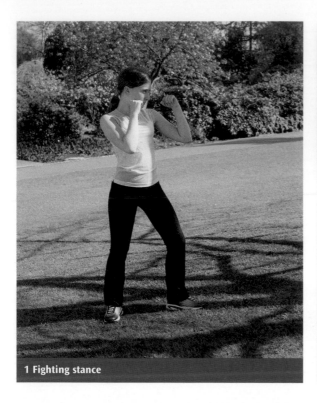

1 Fighting stance

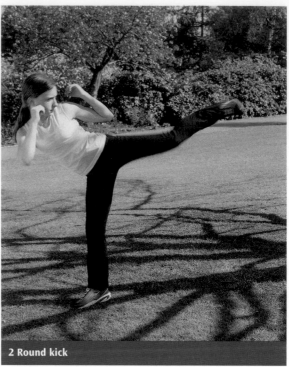

2 Round kick

Exercise 7 – combination

Front-leg round kick

This kick can vary in difficulty from leg to leg depending on the flexibility of your hips. It is perfectly normal for this kick to be harder on one side than the other! Just keep practising. A round kick is essentially the same kick as a roundhouse, but comes off the front leg whereas the roundhouse comes off the back leg.

1 Begin in fighting stance with the right leg behind.

2 Lift and fold the front knee, turning the body completely sideways and pivoting back as you point your knee towards the target. You are now in the chambered position – the knee should be horizontal.

3 Snap the kick out quickly, hitting the target with the lower part of your shin. Snap the leg back to the chambered position and return it immediately to the original fighting stance.

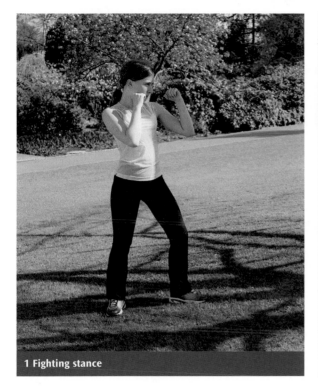

1 Fighting stance

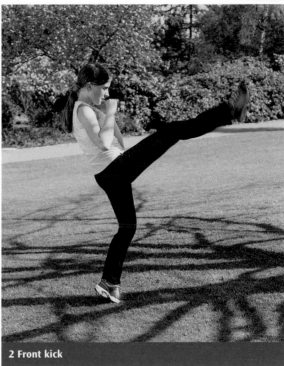

2 Front kick

Front kick–round kick

1 Begin in fighting stance with the right leg behind.

2 Throw a front kick off the rear right leg, dropping it back in the original stance.

3 Now immediately throw a front-leg round kick off the front left leg – you may need to practise this by itself first.

Do
Level one:
right leg behind – 15 combinations
left leg behind – 15 combinations

Level two:
right leg behind – 20 combinations
left leg behind – 20 combinations

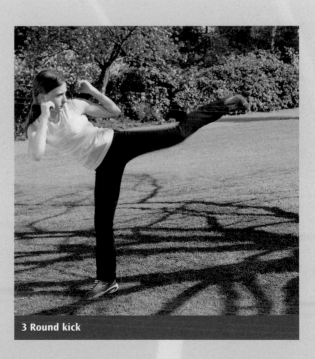

3 Round kick

Exercise 8 – aerobic kicks

Practise this exercise first before you build up the speed.

Side knees

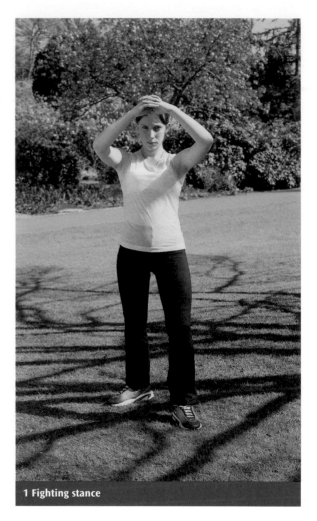

1 Begin in fighting stance with the right leg behind. Make a double-handed grab around the neck of your imaginary opponent, making sure your weight is evenly distributed on both legs.

2 Now shift your weight to the front leg and lift the rear leg, with the knee bent, into a vertical position, with your knee at the side of your body.

3 Pull your hands towards the right side of your body. At the same time, swing the knee – keeping it vertical – into the target area. The striking surface is the meaty part on the inside of the knee.

Do
Level one:
right leg behind – 20 kicks
left leg behind – 20 kicks

Level two:
right leg behind – 30 kicks
left leg behind – 30 kicks

1 Fighting stance

08

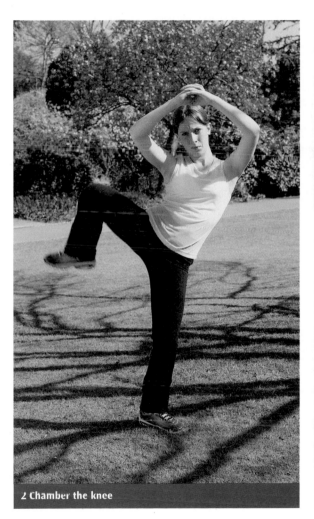

2 Chamber the knee

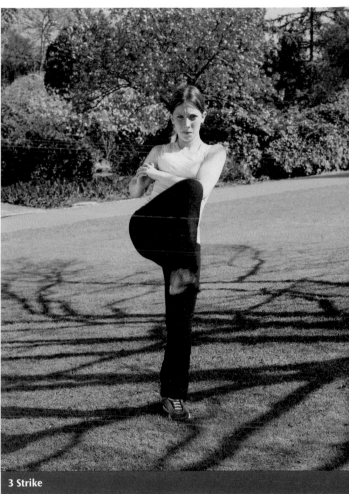

3 Strike

Cool-down and stretch

Now finish your workout with the cool-down section, and spend the last part working through a good, long stretch (see pages 63–67). All your muscles are now loose and warm and in prime condition not only to enjoy but also to benefit from the final stretch.

FAT-BURN CIRCUIT CLASS

From anybody's perspective, Master Martin Ace looks fit; but what not everyone sees is that he works hard at it. After working in the IT industry for 11 years, Martin made his on-going martial-arts hobby into his life's work, which now keeps him busy on a consistent and successful basis. However, it wasn't a sudden decision to change career paths – it took a long, hard thought process. Martin had been studying martial arts since he was 16, first learning sul ki do, then wing chun kung fu, and finally tae kwon do, which he now teaches on a professional basis. Although he was passionate about his martial arts (and not about his IT career), Martin was concerned about how to make his hobby his work. But it was his passion and his belief in how martial arts work as a very effective personal-development tool that swayed his decision. Knowing the positive effects his training had made on his own life committed him to showing others these benefits.

You may find it heartening to hear that, although Martin makes tae kwon do his life, he is not always perfect when it comes to a healthy lifestyle. In fact, he finds it hard to keep off the late-night fast food to which he often succumbs. But his is a success story; he has learned the benefits and the joys of healthy eating, of an active lifestyle and of cross training – he regularly goes running, attends box-a-cise classes, and weight trains whenever he can find the time.

Martin now runs his own classes and teaches on a one-to-one basis in north London. So, what is his advice on how to look for a good martial-arts instructor? 'A great instructor may not be excellent at his or her particular style (at performing the more advanced moves to perfection or in a flashy way). However, a good instructor needs a solid technical knowledge of his or her sport, has to be a good communicator, and must be an excellent motivator. People learn in different ways, so a good instructor (in fact, "teacher" is a better term) must be able to teach in all different manners. Look for a teacher who wants to help you to develop, not cater to his or her own ego or show off!'

The workout

This is a circuit that Martin routinely uses in his tae kwon do class as a basic fitness workout. Circuits are a simple and very effective way of incorporating both resistance work (for body toning and strengthening) with fat-burning cardiovascular exercises. Start by doing a thorough warm-up (see pages 58–62), then move onto the circuit. Spend 30 seconds on each exercise (or 'station', as they are known in circuit classes), then move on immediately to the next. Aim to do each station between 3 and 5 times, depending on the time available and your fitness level. Finish off your workout with a cool-down and stretching routine (see pages 63–67). Aim to be working at 70–75 per cent of your MHR (see page 41), depending on your level of fitness.

Press-ups or three-quarter press-ups

1 Begin on your hands and knees with your hands directly in line with your shoulders and fingers facing forwards. Your arms should be just over shoulder-width apart. For full press-ups, take your legs back so your body is in a straight line and you are resting on your toes. If you like to take less body weight on your arms, use the three-quarter press-ups – for these, work your legs back so you are resting on the fleshy part just above the kneecap (see page 147).

2 Flex your elbows, lowering the chest towards the ground (but not actually reaching the floor), keeping the back straight and the abdominal muscles tight at all times. Straighten up, taking care not to lock your elbows at the top of the move.

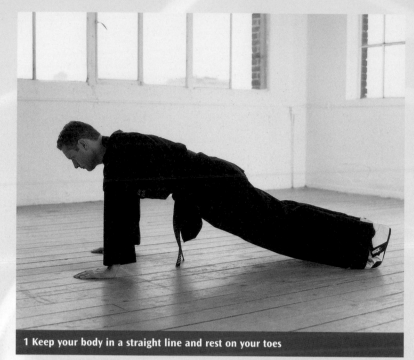

1 Keep your body in a straight line and rest on your toes

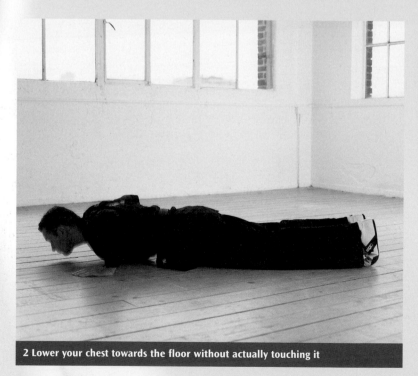

2 Lower your chest towards the floor without actually touching it

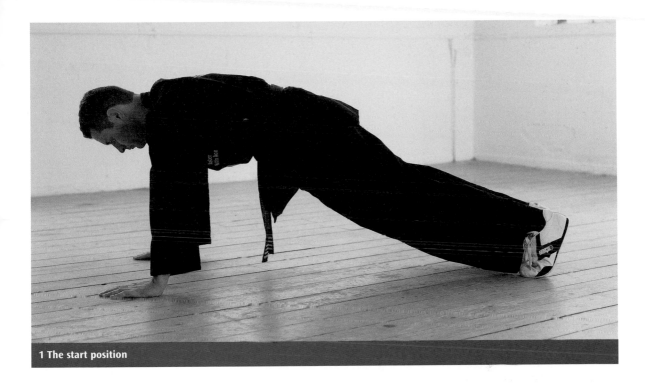

1 The start position

Squat thrusts

1 Place your hands on the floor, shoulder-width apart, with your fingers facing forwards. Take your legs back until your body is almost in a straight line.

2 Jump forwards with both feet, bringing your knees in towards the chest. As soon as you land, jump back to the starting position and repeat. Remember to keep your abdominal muscles tight throughout the move and your bottom low (don't stick it up in the air). To make this exercise easier, use alternate legs one at a time.

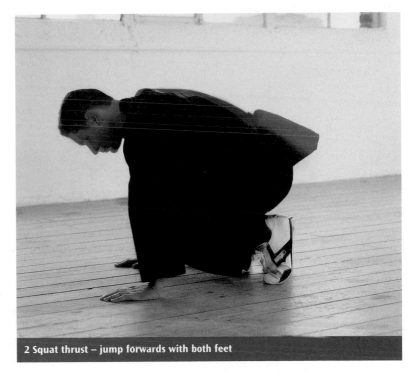

2 Squat thrust – jump forwards with both feet

Crunches

1 Lie on your back with your legs up in the air and feet gently flexed. (To make this exercise easier, drop your ankles down towards your buttocks, keeping your knees upright, and cross your ankles.) Place your fingers at the sides of your head, gently cupping your ears with your hands and allowing your elbows to fall naturally out to the side.

2 Breathing out and keeping your chin off your chest, lift the shoulder blades, shoulders and then head off the floor. Return slowly to the start position.

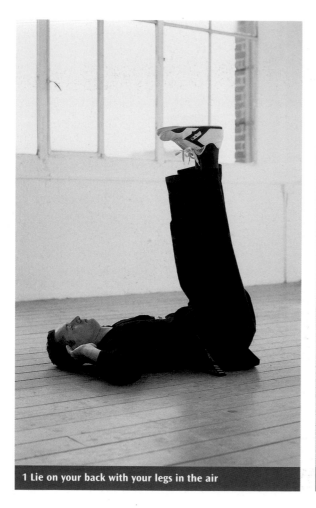

1 Lie on your back with your legs in the air

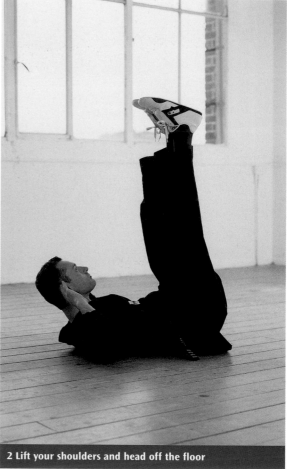

2 Lift your shoulders and head off the floor

Superman

1 Lie on the floor with your arms outstretched in front of you. Keep your nose pointing down to the ground. Now, simultaneously lift your left arm and right leg off the floor. This is not a big move, so try and keep it slow and controlled at all times.

2 Return the arm and leg to the ground and repeat using the right arm and left leg.

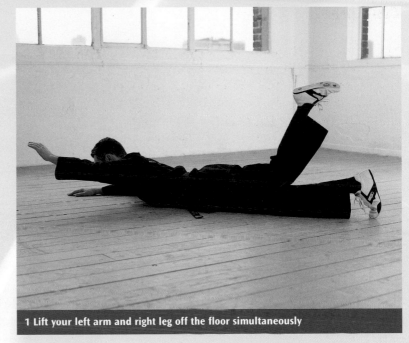

1 Lift your left arm and right leg off the floor simultaneously

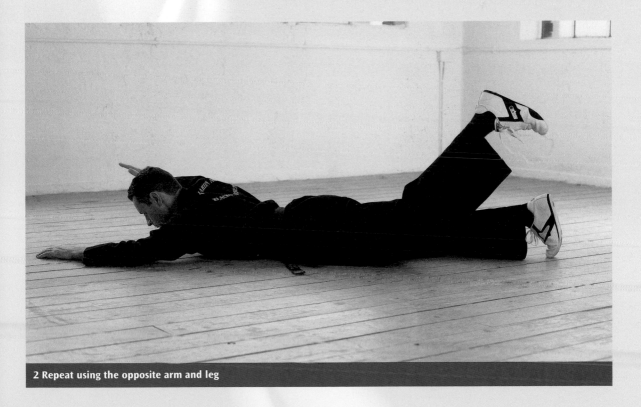

2 Repeat using the opposite arm and leg

Exercise 5

Star jumps

1 Start with your feet hip-width apart and arms by your sides.

2 Jump your feet further apart, landing with your feet flat on the ground and your knees soft. At the same time, take your arms out to the sides and raise them above your head, keeping the elbows bent. Immediately return to the start position and repeat. Alternatively, you can replace this exercise with skipping (see page 48).

Cool-down and stretch

Remember to finish your workout with a thorough cool-down and stretching routine (see pages 63–67).

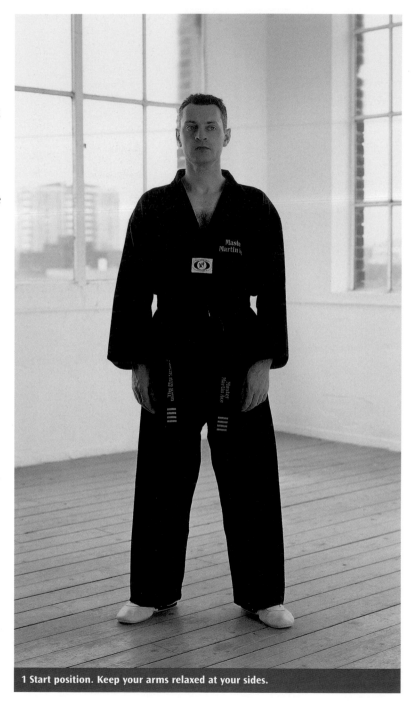

1 Start position. Keep your arms relaxed at your sides.

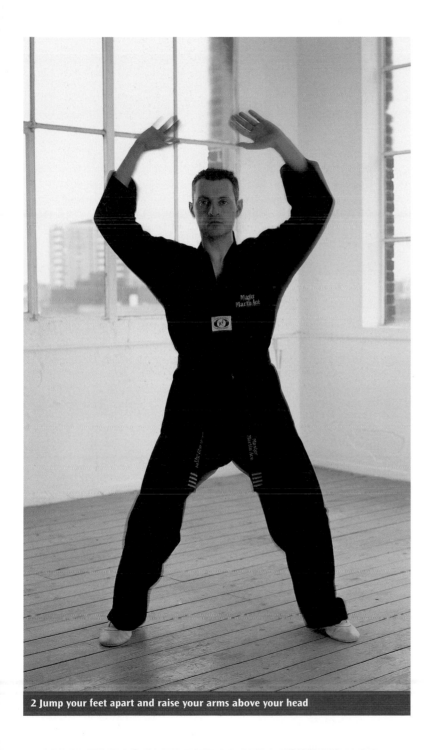

2 Jump your feet apart and raise your arms above your head

ADVANCED WORKOUT

This advanced workout features more intricate combinations of the basic moves as well as introducing a few new ones. To get the most out of the workout, begin with the intermediate workout, then carry on straight through the advanced. However, if you want a simple (yet still advanced) short workout, use the warm-up routine (see pages 58–62), then just use the following exercises. Try to throw the combinations without thinking about them. Move from side to side and back and forth – be light on your feet and ready for anything!

Exercise 1 – combination

Round kick–jab–cross–rear-leg front kick

1 Begin in fighting stance with your right leg behind.

2 Throw a front round kick with your left leg, remembering to pivot back as you point the knee towards the target. Snap the kick out quickly, chamber and then return to your original fighting stance.

3 As you set the leg down, throw a jab.

4 Follow the jab immediately with a cross.

5 As soon as the cross recoils, throw a rear-leg front kick, letting your body move slightly back as the hips move forwards. Snap the kick back, returning to fighting stance.

Do
right leg behind – 25 combinations
left leg behind – 25 combinations

09

This workout is not divided into levels one and two, as I am assuming you now feel you have gained sufficiently in your fitness levels for you to be able to attack this workout and give it your all. However, if you wish to give the workout a try and are unsure about your abilities, cut the repetitions and times down by 50 per cent to begin with. There are also no cardio breaks as such – the aerobic kicks take their place in this workout. You might find at this level that you begin to work out periodically in an 'anaerobic' capacity – i.e. getting out of breath. This is fine, and if you feel comfortable with it, it is a great way for you to begin training.

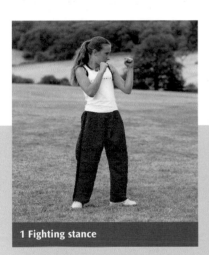

1 Fighting stance

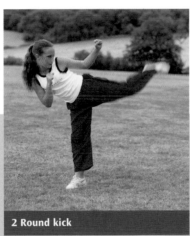

2 Round kick

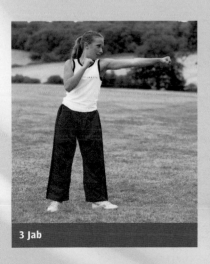

3 Jab

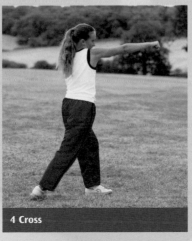

4 Cross

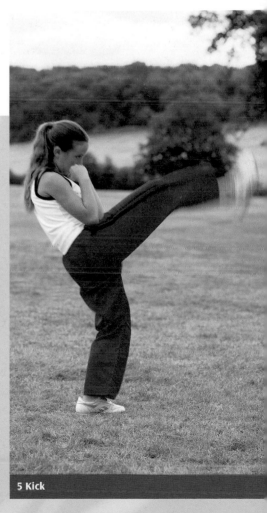

5 Kick

Exercise 2 – aerobic kicks

This is quite a flashy-looking move, more often seen in tae kwon do (the Korean martial art) than in kick-boxing. However, it is a great move to master, looks good and is very aerobic. Don't be put off if you find it hard to begin with – it's all about rhythm and timing. Keep practising – that will be a workout in itself. The aim is for both feet to be off the ground during the kick itself, leaving you with much more scope for the target and height of kick.

Begin by practising this jumping-knees exercise. Start with your legs hip-width apart, knees soft and toes facing forwards. Place your hands either in your regular guard position (as in the fighting stance) or by your sides. Begin lifting your knees as though you were doing regular knee lifts. Now, as one leg begins to travel back towards the floor, use this momentum from the lift to jump into an opposite knee lift. Keep going – the idea is that both feet are off the ground at one point during each knee lift. Remember to land softly by keeping both your knees and ankles flexed and sinking into them, cushioning any impact.

Jumping front kicks (left–right)

1 Begin in fighting stance with your right leg behind.

2 Lift your front (left) knee as quickly as possible.

3 Just before your left foot touches back down on the ground, use the momentum from the lift to raise your back (right) leg to fire a front kick. Do not worry about the height of the kick to begin with; just learn the rhythm and timing of this particular move.

Do
Right leg behind – build up to 50 repetitions

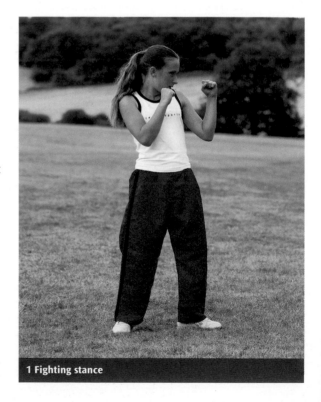

1 Fighting stance

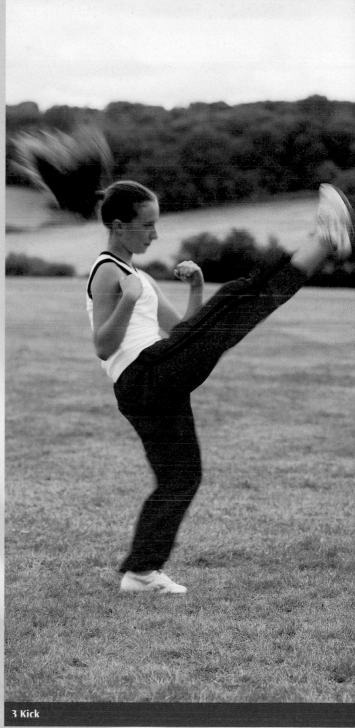

3 Kick

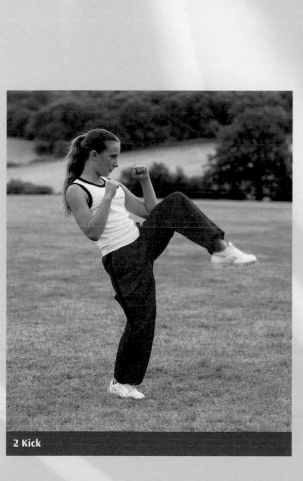

2 Kick

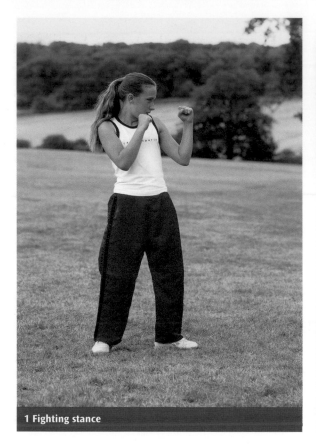

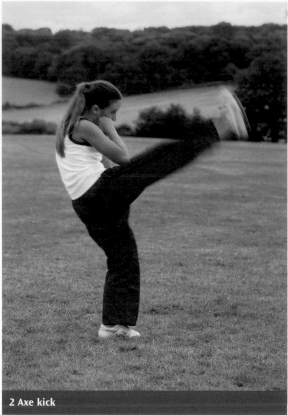

1 Fighting stance

2 Axe kick

Exercise 3 – combination

Axe kick–round kick–jab–cross

1 Begin in fighting stance with the right leg behind.

2 Throw an axe kick with the rear (right) leg. Remember to keep the kicking knee slightly bent and to raise the leg in a slight arc, angling to a point above the target. Chop the kick down, twisting your hips to the right. Drop the leg back to the original fighting stance.

3 Follow up immediately with a left-leg round kick, snapping this kick back and returning to fighting stance.

4 Finish up by moving in on your opponent with a quick jab and cross.

Do
right leg behind – 25 combinations
left leg behind – 25 combinations

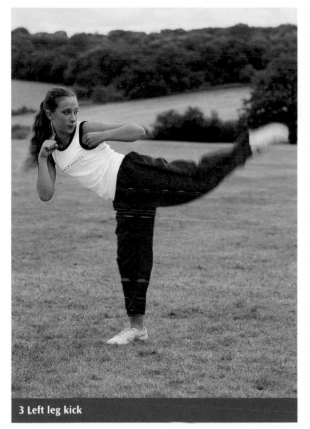

3 Left leg kick

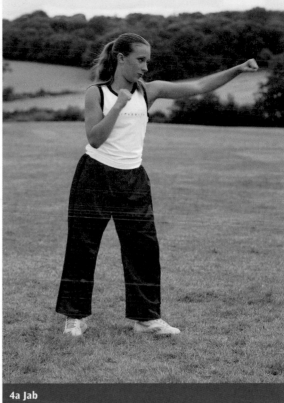

4a Jab

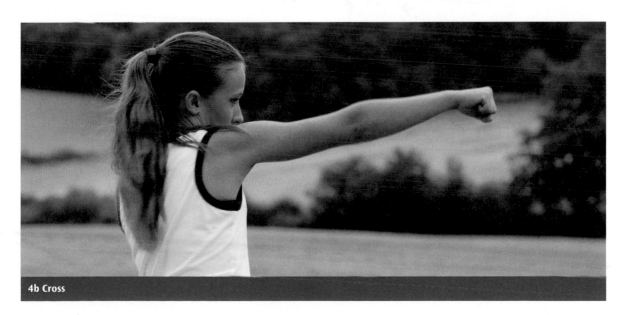

4b Cross

Exercise 4 – aerobic kicks

Jumping front kicks (right–left)

These kicks are a mirror image of the jumping front kicks (left–right) shown on pages 114–115. Begin in fighting stance with your left leg behind. Lift your front right knee as quickly as possible. Just before the right foot touches back down on the ground, use the momentum from the lift to raise your back left leg to fire a front kick. Remember this is all about speed, bounce and timing – so keep practising.

Do
Left leg behind – build up to 50 repetitions

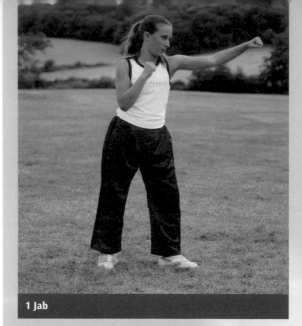
1 Jab

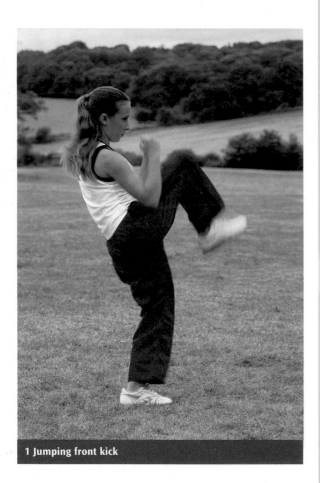
1 Jumping front kick

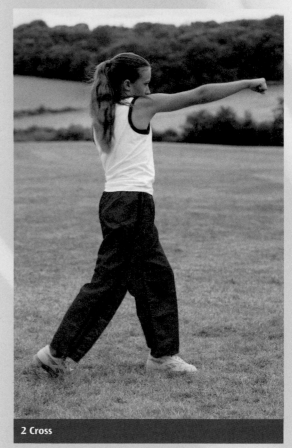
2 Cross

09

Exercise 5 – combination

Jab–cross–rear knee strike–round kick

1 Begin in fighting stance with the right leg behind and throw a left jab.

2 Follow up the jab with a right cross.

3 After the cross recoils, immediately send out a rear knee strike from the back (right) leg. Remember to grab your imaginary opponent around the neck, shifting your weight onto your front leg and, at the same time, shooting the rear knee up.

4 Drop the leg back down into the original stance and immediately follow through with a round kick off the front (left) leg.

Do
right leg behind – 25 combinations
left leg behind – 25 combinations

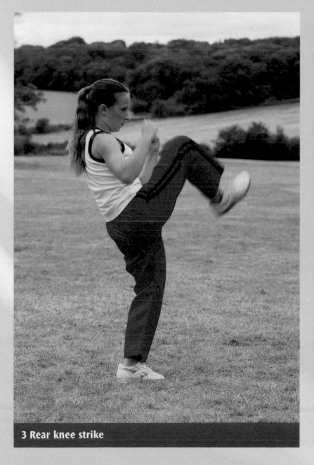

3 Rear knee strike

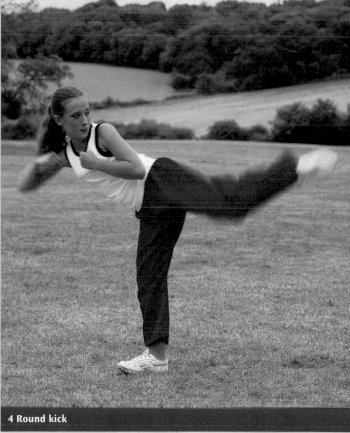

4 Round kick

Exercise 6 – combination

Jab–spinning back fist–cross

1 Begin in fighting stance with your right leg behind. Move in quickly with your left jab.

2 Immediately follow through with a spinning back fist from the right hand. Remember to spin through by turning backwards as quickly as possible, leading with your right shoulder. As you spin, whip the right arm out in a horizontal position, striking the target with the back part of your hand.

3 You will now find yourself in fighting stance with your left leg behind. Finish up by following up with a left-hand cross.

Do
right leg behind – 30 combinations
left leg behind – 30 combinations

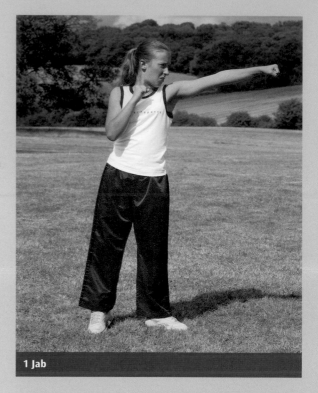

1 Jab

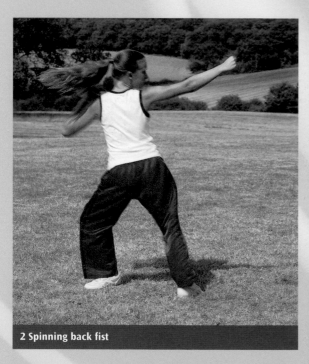

2 Spinning back fist

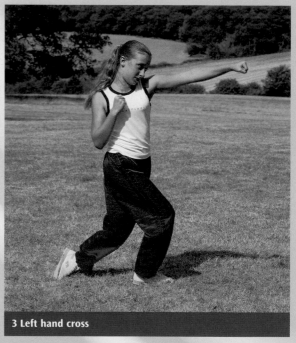

3 Left hand cross

09

Exercise 7 – combination

Overhand

This is a variation of the cross punch. Whereas the cross is fired in a straight line to the face, the overhand curves in a looping motion, aiming towards the side of the jaw or temple.

Begin in fighting stance with your right leg behind. As you fire the punch, the right shoulder twists forward and the left shoulder pulls back. The line of the fist moves in a slight looping motion, the palm of the hand facing down. The punch slides over and down to land on the target. Recoil the arm quickly back to your original stance.

Jab–overhand–body hook

1 Begin in fighting stance with your right leg behind. Fire a jab.

2 Follow the jab by an overhand punch. You may like to practise this move by itself a few times first.

3 Bend deep at the knees, placing your head at your imaginary opponent's chest level. Then deliver a front-hand left hook to their unprotected body. Return to your original stance.

Do

right leg behind – 30 combinations
left leg behind – 30 combinations

Cool-down and stretch

Now finish this workout with a cool-down and spend the last part working through the stretch component (see pages 63–67).

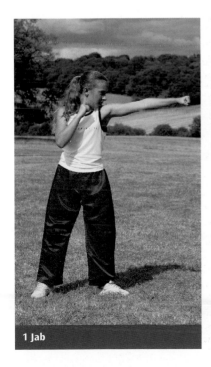

1 Jab

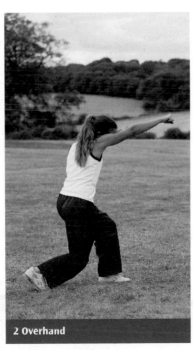

2 Overhand

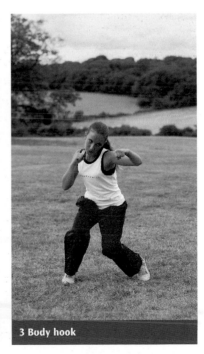

3 Body hook

Moving on

If you find that you work through this (and the other routines) with ease, maybe it's time for you to go beyond the bounds of this book. Why don't you try putting some of your favourite punches and kicks together to create your own combinations? Start by putting two punches or kicks together, then add a third and a fourth to increase the difficulty. You are bound to have your own preferred punches and kicks – they are usually the ones you are good at. However, don't neglect the ones that you find hard. Remember, practice makes perfect and it is a great feeling to master a difficult move.

Pad and bag work

You will have, no doubt, seen kick-boxers and boxers working with a bag. Bag work (as well as working against hand-held pads) is a major part of a professional kick-boxer's workouts. It is important for two reasons. First, it provides resistance. Kicking and punching into the air will give you a great aerobic and toning workout, but actually hitting a bag causes you to work a lot harder (a bit like weight training). Secondly, it gives you the feeling of hitting a live target.

The easiest way to get started is to invest in a freestanding bag for your home and a pair of gloves. These can be bought from most sports suppliers and department stores.

Bear in mind that this is going to be a very different type workout from the ones you have done up to now. You will need to make sure you hit and kick the bag relatively precisely, as it is not as forgiving of poor technique as thin air – so be warned. It is a great workout, though. Not only that, but it will really help you release some tension. Had a bad day? Someone annoyed you? Hit the bag!

There are a number of different ways to work the bag. First, spend some time trying out the various kicks and punches individually, then you can move on. Try working out in rounds. Set a timer for 2 minutes (which is the time of most kick-boxing rounds) and hit the bag continuously for the whole 2 minutes. Take a minute's rest between rounds, but make sure you keep yourself moving – try skipping or jogging around the room. Vary your kicks and punches between speed and power. Tap the bag for some, then give it a wallop for the power attacks. (To get more of an idea of this type of workout, take a look at Kerry-Louise Norbury and Master Cris Janson Piers' workout on pages 24-27.) As always, remember to warm up, cool-down and strecth before and after every workout.

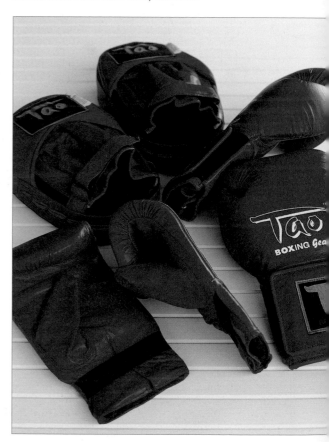

Other equipment

Moving on from the advanced workout, you may wish to try working out using some equipment. Don't be put off by this list – it's not as macho as it sounds. None of these items is required for the workouts in this book, but if you are at all interested in taking the sport of kick-boxing further, you will need to acquire some of the following.

Heavy bag

This is a great piece of equipment if you work out by yourself and you have the space at home (and a good place to hang one). You can use a heavy bag to either kick or punch on. However, be warned, unless you have a very heavy bag (rather hard to hang in a domestic environment) or someone to hold the back of it, it will swing back towards you!

Hand wraps

These are the cheapest piece of equipment you will need and are important for keeping your hands protected. They support the bones in your hands by keeping them tight and compact, while protecting the wrist from the shock of repeated punching onto a hard target. They are made of cotton or gauze and will require washing every now and then. For this you can either use a specific hand-wrap wash bag or just stick them in a washable bag like a pillowcase before putting them in the machine. Don't tumble dry them.

Bag gloves

There are two different types of gloves: bag gloves and sparring gloves. Bag gloves are used during training and have extra padding around the knuckles. It is these you will need first and foremost. They come in various materials, sizes and colours, so it is worth trying on a number of pairs until you find a perfect fit. After finding the best make and size for you, your next question will be what weight you wish to train in. On average, bag gloves weigh 150–350 g (5–12 oz). A lighter glove will do, but most trainers recommend the heavier 350-g (12-oz) glove for beginners, as you get more padding and hence more protection.

Sparring gloves

These gloves are for later on in your training if you decide to begin sparring with other people. Again, they come in different sizes and weights, so it's best to ask your kick-boxing trainer for his or her advice on what would most suit your needs.

Shin pads

These are very popular and, if you have delicate 'girlie' shins as I do, they are well worth getting. They are designed to protect your shins whether you are kicking onto a bag or trying out your kicks on a real person. Make sure they cover your entire shin, extending down to the instep of the foot. Try to get a pair with foot pads (which will protect the top portion of the foot and toes), otherwise you can buy them separately.

Focus mitts

These are the round pads that your partner or trainer wears on their hands to help you work on your boxing techniques. They are made by a number of different manufacturers and come in different qualities. Try to avoid buying a cheap flimsy pair; as with most of this equipment, it is worthwhile buying the sturdiest and best quality you can afford.

Thai pads and kicking shields

Both of these pieces of equipment are for you to practise your kicking techniques on. Thai pads (not surprisingly, originating in Thailand) are thick heavy-duty rectangular pads 45–50 cm (18–20 in) by 20–25 cm (8–10 in). The thick padding is designed to protect the person holding the pad, which is held by straps and handles sewn onto the back. Kicking shields are bigger and are great for practising your kicks at full power.

KICK-BOX CLASS

KERRY NORBURY & CRIS JANSON-PIERS

If there was ever a more unlikely potential world kick-boxing champion, I would be amazed, for Kerry-Louise Norbury is one of the most quietly modest and unassuming kick-boxing champions I have had the pleasure to meet. At the age of 22 she trains every day and is multi-English and multi-British Freestyle Karate Champion. She was placed second in the War of the World competition, holding a silver medal, and after competing in the world championships in Paris in October 2003 is currently seeded number 7 at world-level full-contact kick-boxing. She is a qualified instructor, coach and referee and is also the highest ranked female in the British Freestyle Karate & Kickboxing Organization, which all in all is not bad for someone who wanted to take up horse riding instead!

At the age of seven, Kerry-Louise found herself being bullied at school. Though wishing to go horse riding as a hobby, her mother insisted she took up martial arts instead, at least until she had learned to protect herself. It didn't come naturally in the first few months, but she managed to win her first competition in her first year of training and has gone from strength to strength ever since.

Her trainer and partner is Cris Janson-Piers, who has 27 years of martial-arts experience behind him. Initially in the Royal Signals and Military police, he began his martial-arts career in the combined services judo team before moving on to incorporate a myriad of martial-art styles and skills from freestyle karate to kick-boxing.

These days Cris divides his time between teaching, coaching and his own training, and also runs a security and close-protection company. He says: 'I enjoy the results personal training gives, it is an accelerated system and gives a great sense of achievement to both client and coach. Individual needs can be catered for a lot more easily on a one-to-one basis, whether it is diet or exercise. However, I must say though that normal group lessons should not be underestimated! You get out of them what you put in, and the friendly atmosphere and social aspect of an organized club are excellent.'

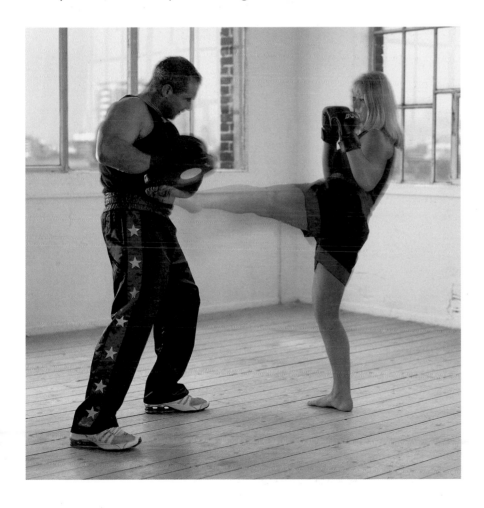

Kick-box Class: Kerry Norbury and Cris Janson-Piers

The workout

To get some idea of what it's like to train with equipment, a partner and in a club situation, take a look at this workout that Cris and Kerry are doing.

Cris first gets Kerry-Louise to do a couple of 2-minute rounds of 'pedal and jab' working onto his hand-held focus mitts. Kerry works in what is called a speed-ball motion on the mitts. This action mimics working on a speed-ball – this is the suspended leather ball you will associate with a classic boxer workout. A speed-ball is like skipping for the hands, helping build speed, timing, rhythm and hand–eye coordination. You need to be quick, though, since the ball ricochets back and forth as you hit it, leaving you no time to think, and it – unlike Cris holding the focus mitts – won't mind giving you a quick thump in the face if you are not paying attention!

In between each exercise, Cris advocates one minute of skipping, and then it is on to the next exercise. For Kerry-Louise it is a two-minute round of kicks onto the pads. This time it is a combination of straight-leg round kicks, changing the leading kicking leg after the 2 minutes and repeating.

Next is another 2-minute bout of punching, followed by a jab, cross, bob and weave, with Cris applying the focus mitts in a hooking motion over Kerry-Louise's head to simulate her potential opponent's method of attack. Bobbing and weaving is simply a way to make you a more elusive target by ducking your opponent's attack. You need to remember two things. First, keep your hands up when ducking – this way, if you misjudge the attack, your hands are there to block. Secondly, if your first reaction is to bend forward at the waist, resist it. Bending down in this way can throw you off balance – instead, bend at the knees whilst keeping your chest up, squatting down to avoid the attack, but not taking your head below waist level.

Another combination of kicks onto the large hand-held pad is a double front-leg push kick followed up immediately by a reverse-leg round kick. Think of a 'push' kick being

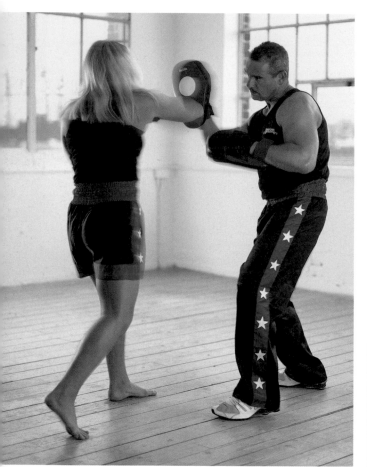

> **IMPORTANT**
>
> Please don't try this at home! Training on to pads requires expert tuition. If you'd like to take your kick-boxing to this level, you need to have qualified experienced instruction, either on a one-to-one basis or as part of a class. You will learn to use training aids and equipment, such as the gloves and pads (there is as much as skill to holding the pads as to using them).

simply that: you are pushing (with a thrust of power) your opponent away from you. Chambering from the classic front-kick stance, the push kick uses power from the hips the moment the ball of the foot makes impact with the target. Following this up with the round kick makes a very powerful combination indeed.

Finally Kerry-Louise finishes off with a burst of energy and power – pummelling away on the large pad whilst jogging on the spot. This might look easy, but by the end of this workout you will fight to find every last ounce of strength and energy – exactly what this designed to do. Cris finishes off this particular workout with a couple of minutes' shadow-boxing then moves into a cool-down routine, and the last minutes are spent stretching out every major muscle group.

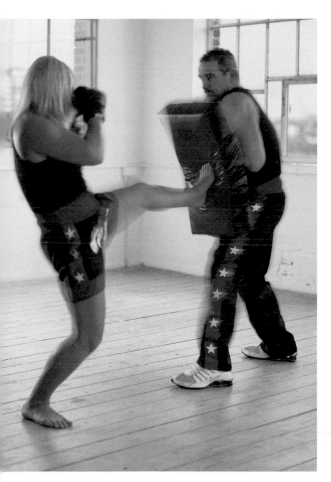
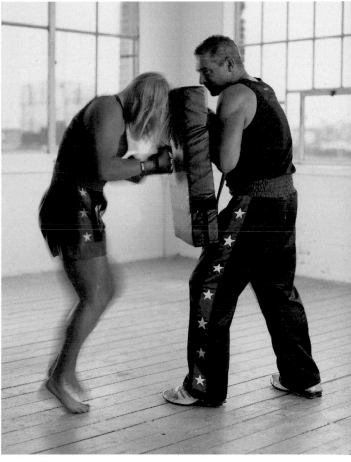

CHAPTER TEN

QUICK WORKOUT

This is a very short and simple workout combining both kick-boxing and basic resistance exercises (using hand weights, see page 48). It is designed to work the whole body in a minimum amount of time. Do not skimp on your warm-up, cool-down and stretches, though – they are as important as ever.

In order to do this workout, you will need to be familiar with all the basic moves in the beginners' workout (pages 76–85). Two levels are provided – choose the one that suits you.

A NOTE ABOUT SETS AND REPS

Reps (or repetitions) are the number of times you are asked to do an exercise. For level one exercises, you are asked to do a specific number of reps. For some of the level two exercises, you are asked to do two sets of reps. You must rest for a minimum of 30 seconds (and a maximum of one minute) between sets to get optimum benefit. So, do the required reps, rest for 30–60 seconds, then repeat.

Exercise 1

Jab–cross–front kick

1 Begin in fighting stance with your right leg behind. Throw a jab with the lead (left) hand.

2 Follow up with a right-handed cross.

3 As the cross recoils, throw a front kick off the rear (right) leg.

Do
Level one:
right leg behind – 20 combinations
left leg behind – 20 combinations

Level two:
right leg behind – 30 combinations
left leg behind – 30 combinations

Cardio break

Either skip with or without a rope. However, using a rope is a great way to burn calories. Don't try to jump too high, and keep your knees and ankles soft.

Or jog on the spot or, preferably, around the room. Keep your knees and ankles soft. Use your arms to pump gently backwards and forwards, keeping your elbows softly flexed.

Do 30–60 seconds

Exercise 2

Squats and lateral raises

1 Holding your hand weights, stand with your feet one-and-half times hip-width apart, your bottom tucked under and shoulders back and down.

2 Take your arms out to your sides up to shoulder height, palms facing downwards and elbows slightly bent at all times. As you lift your arms, squat down. Do not squat any lower than the line of your knees and make sure your knees travel in line with your toes. Return to the start position.

Do
Level one: one set of 16 reps
Level two: two sets of 16 reps

Cardio break – Skipping or jogging

Do
30–60 seconds

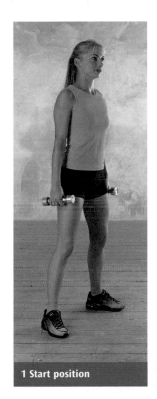
1 Start position

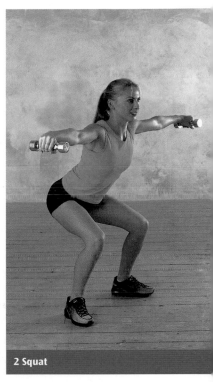
2 Squat

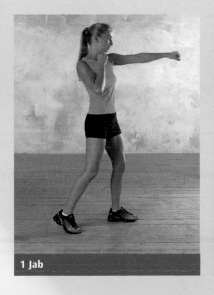
1 Jab

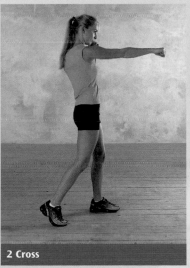
2 Cross

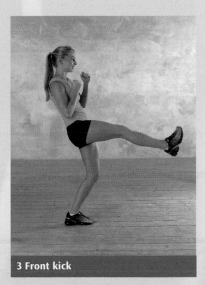
3 Front kick

Exercise 3

Hook–hook–roundhouse

1 Begin in fighting stance with your right leg behind. Throw a double hook, first punching with the front (left) arm.

2 Complete the double hook by following up immediately with a right hook.

3 As you finish the second punch, throw a roundhouse kick off your back (right) leg. Return to the original stance.

Do
Level one:
right leg behind – 20 combinations
left leg behind – 20 combinations
Level two:
right leg behind – 30 combinations
left leg behind – 30 combinations

Cardio break – Skipping or jogging

Do 30–60 seconds

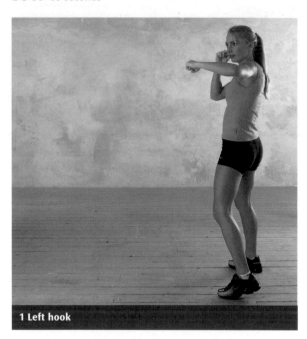
1 Left hook

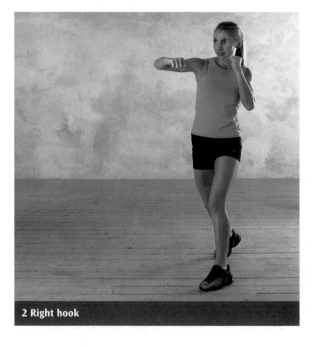
2 Right hook

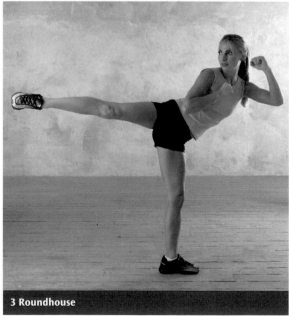
3 Roundhouse

Exercise 4

Lunges and pec deck

1 Start with your feet hip width apart and toes facing forwards. Holding your hand weights, lift your arms out at right angles to the sides of your body, with your elbows flexed upwards. Try to keep your elbows at shoulder height.

2 Now step forwards with the left leg so both knees bend to a right angle as the body is lowered. At the same time, squeeze your forearms together, keeping the elbows high. Keep your body upright with your feet hip-width apart. As you drive back with the leading leg, take your arms back to the start position. Repeat on the other leg, again squeezing the forearms together.

Do
Level one: one set of 16 reps
Level two: two sets of 16 reps

Cool-down and stretch
Finish your workout with a cool-down and stretching routine (see pages 63–67).

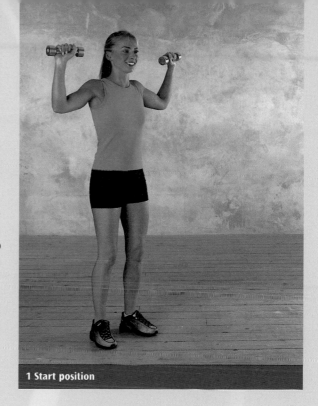

1 Start position

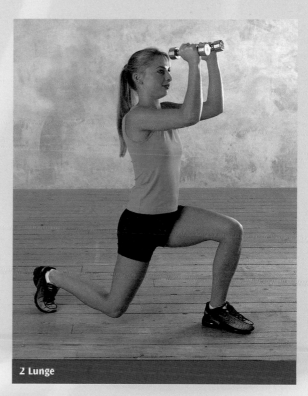

2 Lunge

TROUBLESHOOTING

We all have different areas of our bodies that we would like to improve. The kick-boxing workouts are going to help you lose excess body fat and give you an all-over improved tone. However, if you wish to do that little bit extra, here are some tips for the top six areas that most of us would wish to improve upon.

You can add these individual short workouts to the end of your kick-boxing routine (after the cool-down but before the stretch) or do them by themselves. If this is the case, please make sure you follow the general safe-exercise principles – warm up first for at least 5 minutes, do your chosen workout and finish off with a stretch.

You will need some equipment for these workouts: a mat, a resistance band and some hand weights (see page 48 for options). Choose level one or two, depending on the intensity of the workout you're after. Remember that you need to rest for 30–60 seconds between each set of reps you are asked to do for an exercise (see page 44).

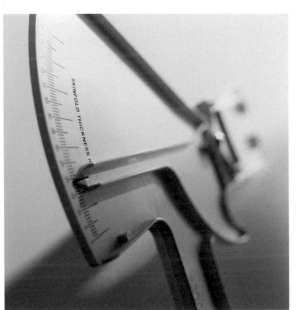

Bottom workout

Though your bottom muscles are particularly large in comparison to the rest of the body, they do firm and tone quite easily given the right combination of exercises and patience. Spend time, during the entire workout, thinking about keeping your bottom muscles squeezed and working hard – it really will make a difference.

Heel press

1 Lie on your back with your left foot flat on the floor and your right knee pulled into your chest. Hold one end of a resistance band in each hand and loop the middle around the bottom of your right foot. Stretch the band tight and press your shoulder blades and elbows into the mat.

2 With your foot flexed, press your right leg out, away from your hands, without locking the knee. Return to the start position and repeat.

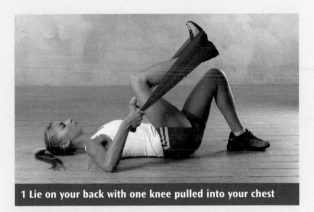

1 Lie on your back with one knee pulled into your chest

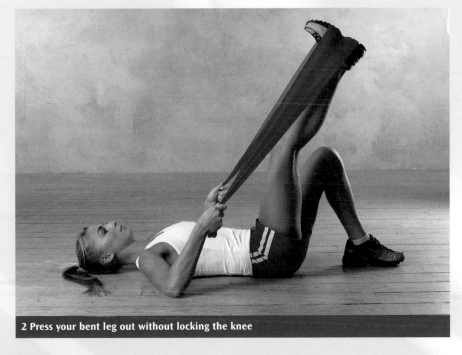

2 Press your bent leg out without locking the knee

Do
Level one: one set of 12–16 reps on each leg
Level two: two sets of 12–16 reps on each leg

Side kick

1 Lie on your right side with your head resting in your right hand and your bottom leg bent for support. Loop a resistance band around the middle of your left foot and grasp both ends in your left hand (draw the band under your left knee, not over it).

2 Keeping the upper body strong and lifted (don't let your shoulder blades sink into the floor), flex your left foot and press the leg out, without locking the knee. At the same time as you press the leg out, lift it so your foot is slightly higher than your hip. Return to the start position.

Do

Level one: one set of 12–16 reps on each side
Level two: two sets of 12–16 reps on each side

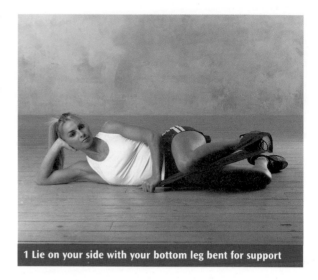

1 Lie on your side with your bottom leg bent for support

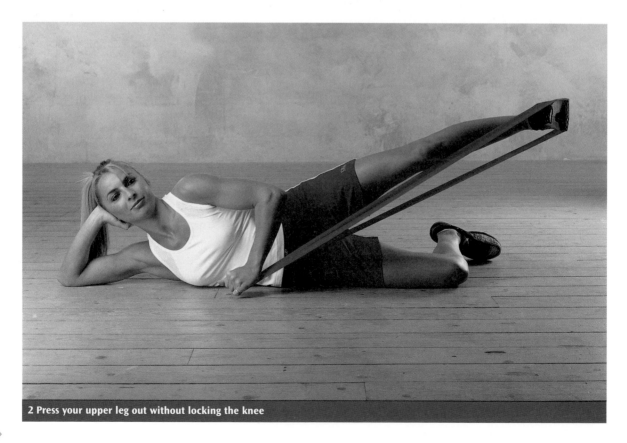

2 Press your upper leg out without locking the knee

11

Glute raises

1 Begin on all fours, resting on your forearms. Keep a straight back and tighten your abdominal muscles to help support your back. Extend your left leg and flex the foot.

2 Keeping your back still, lift the left leg up, squeezing your bottom muscles as you do so. Return the foot slowly to the floor and repeat. Try not to sink into your supporting hip.

Do
Level one: one set of 12–16 reps on each leg
Level two: two sets of 12 16 reps on each leg

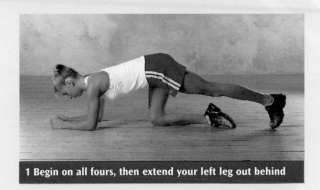
1 Begin on all fours, then extend your left leg out behind

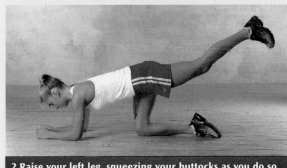
2 Raise your left leg, squeezing your buttocks as you do so

Bottom lift

1 Lie on your back with your feet flat against the floor and arms at your sides with the palms facing down.

2 Tucking your pelvis up, slowly lift your bottom a few inches off the floor. Holding this position, contract your abdominals; press your heels into the floor, and now raise your hips off the floor, too, so you are lifting up another inch. Hold for four counts, then lower your bottom slowly to the floor.

Do
Level one: one set of 12–16 reps
Level two: two sets of 12–16 reps

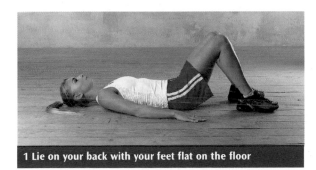
1 Lie on your back with your feet flat on the floor

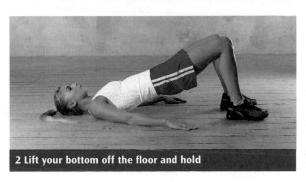
2 Lift your bottom off the floor and hold

Thigh workout

Though you should find kick-boxing to be a great leg and bottom workout in itself, sometimes a little extra care and attention can make all the difference. The following exercises, though concentrating on the thigh area, will have the added bonus of working your bottom too! As always, remember to warm up, cool down and stretch with every workout (see pages 63–67).

Lunges

1 Begin with your legs hip-width apart and your toes facing directly forwards.

2 Step forward with the right leg a sufficient distance to enable both knees to bend to a right angle as the body is lowered. Keep the body upright and the feet hip-width apart (this helps you balance). Look forwards and slightly down. Now drive back with the right leg to the start position and repeat on the other leg.

Do
Level one: one set of 12–16 reps
Level two: two sets of 12–16 reps

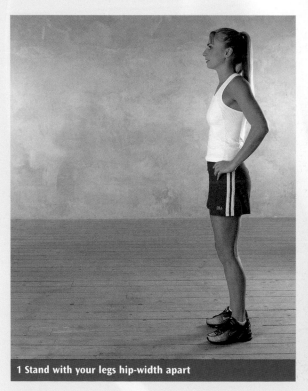

1 Stand with your legs hip-width apart

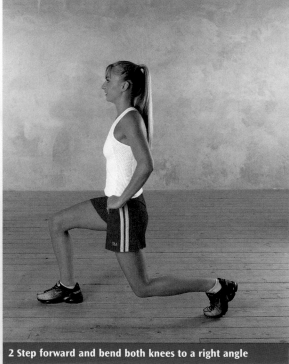

2 Step forward and bend both knees to a right angle

11

Straight leg lifts

1 Lie on your right side with your right arm supporting your neck and head and your left arm in front providing some support for the body. Your hip, knee and upper body should form one line, with the lower leg bent. Lengthen out through the top left leg, gently flexing the foot. The leg should be straight but not locked at the knee joint.

2 Now lift the left leg up as high as feels comfortable, making sure you keep your abdominals tight throughout the exercise. Return the leg slowly to the start position and repeat.

Do
Level one: one set of 12–16 reps on each side
Level two: two sets of 12–16 reps on each side

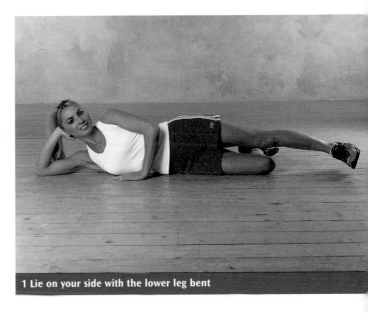
1 Lie on your side with the lower leg bent

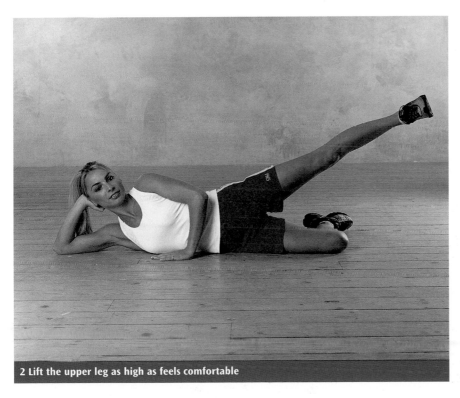
2 Lift the upper leg as high as feels comfortable

Inside thigh

1 Lie on your right side, supporting yourself on your elbows. Keep your left foot flat on the floor behind your right knee. Try to lengthen out through the right leg, stretching it out as far as possible, but keeping a slight bend at the knee. Ensure that the inner thigh of your right leg is turned to the ceiling.

2 Keeping the right foot relaxed, lift the leg towards the ceiling, maintaining the turnout at the hips. Return to the start position and repeat.

Do
Level one: one set of 12–16 reps on each side
Level two: two sets of 12–16 reps on each side

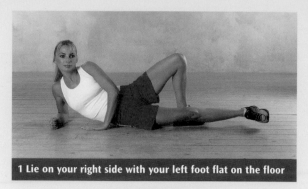
1 Lie on your right side with your left foot flat on the floor

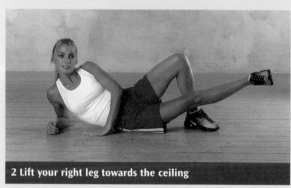
2 Lift your right leg towards the ceiling

Hip opener

1 Lie on your side with your legs bent in front of you (your thighs should be at 90˚ to your torso and your lower leg at 90˚ to your thighs). As you look down towards your knees, you should just be able to see your toes.

2 Now, keeping your feet together and your abdominals

tight, open your thighs as far as possible, hinging at the hips and feet. Return the upper leg slowly to the start and repeat.

Do
Level one: one set of 12–16 reps on each side
Level two: two sets of 12–16 reps on each side

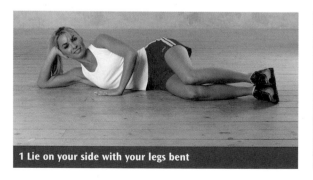
1 Lie on your side with your legs bent

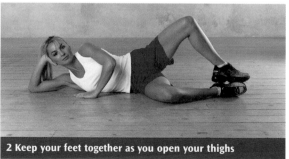
2 Keep your feet together as you open your thighs

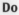

Abdominal workout

Most people (and especially women) dream of having a flat tummy, and you'll be pleased to know that the dream is not beyond your grasp. However, it is the unfortunate truth that this is where most women lay down excess fat, hiding any muscle tone they may have. This is simply Mother Nature's way of facilitating childbirth – her aim being that, even if you are starving, you will still have enough fat supplies to maintain pregnancy. Don't be put off, though. Follow this abdominal workout and keep up the good work with the fat-burning exercise – your tummy muscles will soon begin to look sleeker and more toned.

Sit-ups

1 Lie on the floor with your back flat, knees bent and feet flat on the floor. Keep your feet relatively close to your bottom so that you are resting firmly on your tail bone with your spine in a neutral position. Keep your feet and knees hip-width apart. Gently cup your ears with your hands, letting your elbows fall naturally to the sides.

2 Lift your body up using your abdominals, so you raise your head, shoulders and then shoulder blades off the floor. Curl up slowly, breathing out as you do so to aid muscle contraction. Lower yourself slowly back down.

Do
Level one: one set of 12–16 reps
Level two: two sets of 12–16 reps

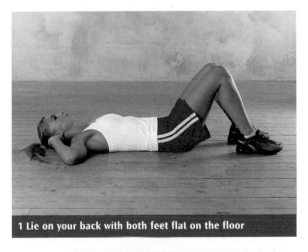

1 Lie on your back with both feet flat on the floor

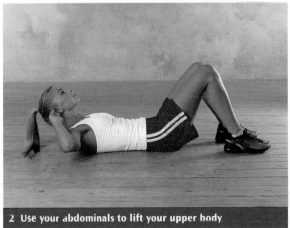

2 Use your abdominals to lift your upper body

Back extensions

1 Lie on your front and place your hands in the small of your back.

2 Keeping your bottom and thighs relaxed, and your nose and chest pointing down towards the ground, lift your chest off the ground. Return slowly to the ground and repeat.

Do
Level one: one set of 12–16 reps
Level two: two sets of 12–16 reps

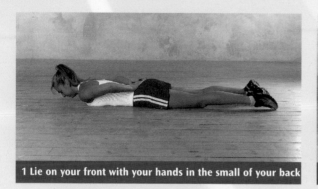
1 Lie on your front with your hands in the small of your back

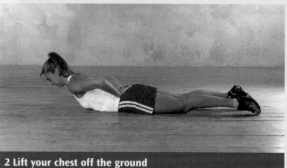
2 Lift your chest off the ground

Heel touch

1 Lie on your back with your knees over your hips and your lower legs parallel to the floor. Make sure your back is firmly pressed into the ground and your spine is in a neutral position.

2 Slowly lower one leg down, dropping the heel to the floor. Lift the leg slowly back up, making sure your spine remains in the neutral position. Repeat with the other leg. Make sure you do this exercise slowly and with control at all times.

Do
Level one: one set of 12–16 reps
Level two: two sets of 12–16 reps

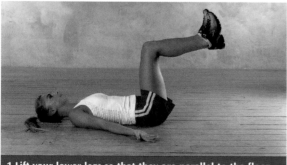
1 Lift your lower legs so that they are parallel to the floor

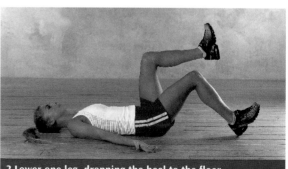
2 Lower one leg, dropping the heel to the floor

Sit up and twist

1 Lie on the floor on your back and press your lower back into the floor, making sure your spine is in a neutral position. Gently cup your ears with your hands, letting your elbows fall naturally out to the sides. Put your right ankle over the left knee, resting on the fleshy part of upper knee.

2 Keeping your lower body as still as possible, take your left shoulder towards the right knee. Hold momentarily, making sure both hips remain firmly on the floor, then return slowly to the start position.

Do

Level one: one set of 12–16 reps on each side
Level two: two sets of 12–16 reps on each side

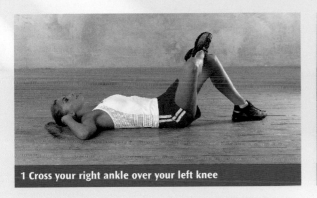

1 Cross your right ankle over your left knee

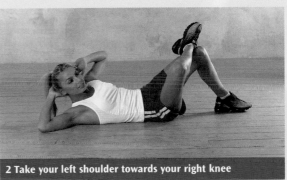

2 Take your left shoulder towards your right knee

The Plank

Begin on your hands and knees with your hands under your shoulders, and knees under hips. Walk back until your legs are straight and you are balancing on your toes with your feet together. Keep your arms straight (but not locked) and your shoulders back and down. Hold for a count of 5 breaths, then release.

Do

Level one: one set of 12–16 reps
Level two: two sets of 12–16 reps

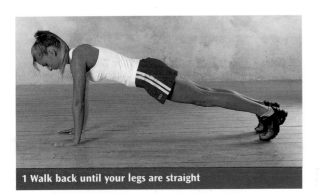

1 Walk back until your legs are straight

Arm workout

Often there comes a point in our lives when our upper arms take on what I call a 'bat-wing' appearance. Luckily, it's easy to restore their tone with the following workout. You'll need your hand weights (see page 48) for this routine, and remember to warm-up, cool-down and stretch before and after your workout (see Chapter Five).

Lying tricep extensions

1 Lie flat on the floor (or on a bench or step), making sure your back is firmly pressed down and your abdominal muscles are tight. Using hand weights, stretch your arms above you, so they are positioned directly above your shoulders.

2 Lock your wrists and keep the upper arms fixed vertically. You should flex from the elbows only. Lower the weights carefully towards your forehead and then extend the arms again until they are straight but not locked.

Do
Level one: one set of 12–16 reps
Level two: two sets of 12–16 reps

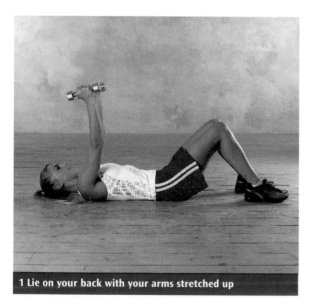

1 Lie on your back with your arms stretched up

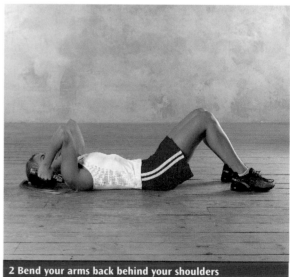

2 Bend your arms back behind your shoulders

11

Bicep curl

1 Stand with your feet one-and-a-half times hip-width apart, knees soft and body upright. Holding onto your hand weights, fix your upper arms into the sides of your body.

2 Curl the weights up towards your armpits, keeping your elbows fixed into the side of your body. Then lower the weights slowly until your arms are straight but not locked.

Do
Level one: one set of 12–16 reps
Level two: two sets of 12–16 reps

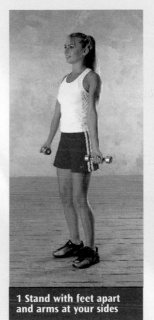
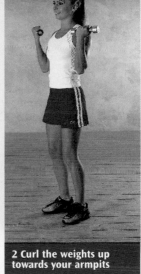

1 Stand with feet apart and arms at your sides

2 Curl the weights up towards your armpits

Hammer-head curls

1 Stand with your feet one-and-a-half times hip-width apart, knees soft and body upright. Holding your hand weights, place your hands to the side of your thighs, palms facing in. Lock your upper arms into the side of your body.

2 Now curl the weights alternately up towards your shoulders. Make sure you do not lock your elbow joints at any point. Keep the move slow and continuous.

Do
Level one: one set of 12–16 reps
Level two: two sets of 12–16 reps

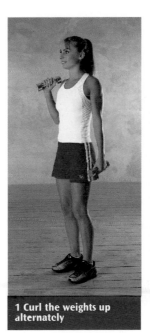
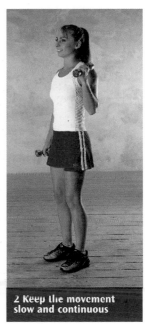

1 Curl the weights up alternately

2 Keep the movement slow and continuous

Tricep kickbacks

1 Stand with your feet hip-width apart in front of a wall or a stable chair. Place your right hand on the wall or chair for support; step back with your left leg and bend slightly forwards. Lift your left elbow back so it is in line with your shoulder, tucking the hand weight in towards your armpit.

2 Now lift your left hand back until your arm is straight out behind you. Make sure you do not lock out your left elbow joint. Return the hand weight slowly towards your armpit, following the original path.

Do

Level one: one set of 12–16 reps on each arm
Level two: two sets of 12–16 reps on each arm

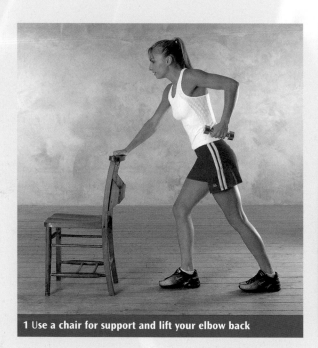

1 Use a chair for support and lift your elbow back

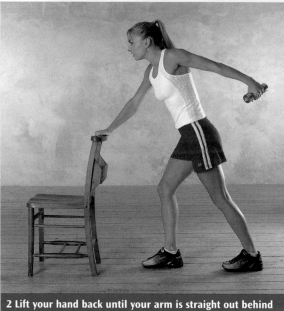

2 Lift your hand back until your arm is straight out behind

Chest workout

Because women's breasts are composed mainly of fatty tissue and contain no muscle, exercise alone will not change the size of your bust. However, you can give the impression of your breasts being pert and firm by training the pectoral muscles which surround the breasts themselves. On a preventative note, it is very important to make sure you wear a good sports bra while exercising. This workout is not designed for women alone – many men can find themselves with the same problems in the chest area, so these exercises will help firm up either sex. You may like to combine this workout with the upper-back workout – together they'll have a fantastic body-toning effect. Remember to warm-up, cool down and stretch with every workout (see Chapter Five). You will need your hand weights for this routine.

Tricep dips

1 Sit on the edge of a stable chair with your legs bent and feet flat on the floor, hip-width apart. Place your hands on either side of your bottom with the fingers facing forwards and hold onto the chair. Now shuffle your weight onto your straight arms (try to keep your arms straight but not locked out through the elbow joint).

2 Keeping your back straight and your abdominal muscles tight, lower yourself towards the floor by flexing at the elbows. Keep your back as close to the chair as possible. Dip down until your arms are at 45°, then straighten up, taking care not to lock the elbows at the top of the move.

Do
Level one: one set of 12–16 reps
Level two: two sets of 12–16 reps

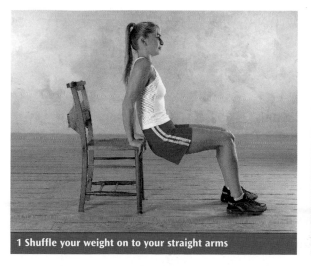
1 Shuffle your weight on to your straight arms

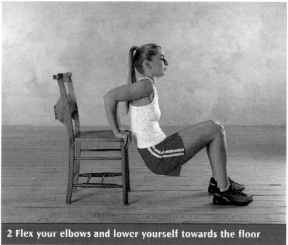
2 Flex your elbows and lower yourself towards the floor

Pec deck

This is one of those exercises that looks deceptively simple but, when it comes down to it, isn't! This is because the smaller shoulder muscles are having to work very hard in order for you to hold those arms (and weights) up. If you find this too hard, try doing it without the weights to begin with.

1 You can do this exercise either seated or standing. Using hand weights, take your arms out so your elbows are level your shoulders, and your lower arms point upwards. Keep your back straight and abdominal muscles tight.

2 Now squeeze your forearms towards each other, keeping your elbows high. Return to the start position.

Do
Level one: one set of 12–16 reps
Level two: two sets of 12–16 reps

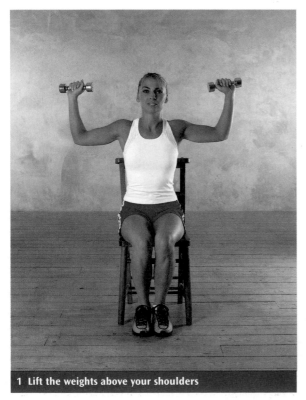

1 Lift the weights above your shoulders

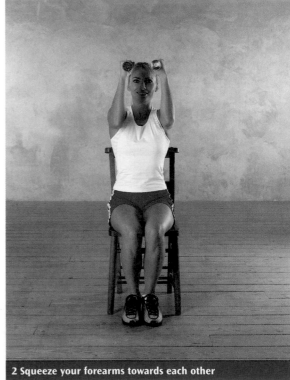

2 Squeeze your forearms towards each other

Press-ups

1 Start on all fours with your knees in line with your hips, and hands in line with your shoulders. Your back should be straight and your abdominals tight. Shuffle your legs back until you are resting on the fleshy apart just above your kneecap and then cross your ankles.

2 Flex at the elbows to lower the head and chest towards the ground in a slow, controlled manner. Straighten up, taking care not to lock out the elbows at the top of the move.

Do
Level one: one set of 12–16 reps
Level two: two sets of 12–16 reps

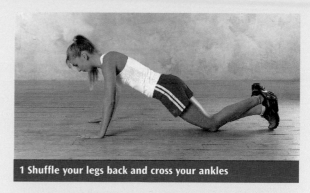
1 Shuffle your legs back and cross your ankles

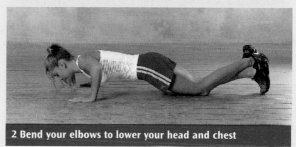
2 Bend your elbows to lower your head and chest

Pull-overs

1 Lie on your back on the floor with your knees bent and feet flat on the floor. Hold one hand weight in both hands and straighten your arms up, in line with your shoulders, keeping a slight bend at the elbows.

2 Keeping the same angle in the elbows, take the weight back and behind your head. Lower the weight in a slow, controlled manner, taking care not to arch your back. Return slowly to the start position.

Do
Level one: one set of 12–16 reps
Level two: two sets of 12–16 reps

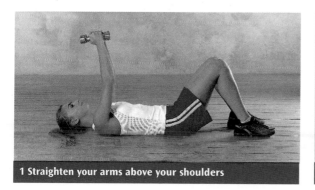
1 Straighten your arms above your shoulders

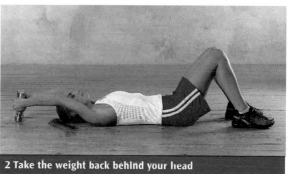
2 Take the weight back behind your head

Upper-back workout

The upper back is one of those trouble spots that creeps up on you, simply because it is not an area you are aware of on a daily basis. However, whether it be an unflattering photograph or just the fact that your flesh is slowly creeping over your bra line, it can come as quite a shock! The great advantage of toning this muscle group is that it will give you a very flattering silhouette; by re-shaping the upper back, you can make your waist look smaller. Since it is very important to maintain a balanced workout, it is advisable to do this workout in conjunction with the chest workout.

You will need a resistance band and hand weights for this workout. And, as always, remember to warm up, cool down and stretch (see Chapter Five).

Seated row

1 Sit on the floor with your legs out in front of you. Wrap a resistance band around the base of your feet and shuffle backwards until your legs are straight, but not locked. Your body should be upright or leaning slightly back, and your arms should be straight.

2 Keeping your abdominals tight, back straight, and maintaining the angle at your hips, pull the band towards your lower chest, leading the movement with your elbows. Keep your wrists firm and avoid any tendency to flex the wrist at the end of the movement. Straighten your arms out slowly until they are straight, but don't lock the elbow joint. Repeat, keeping the movement slow and continuous.

Do
Level one: one set of 12–16 reps
Level two: two sets of 12–16 reps

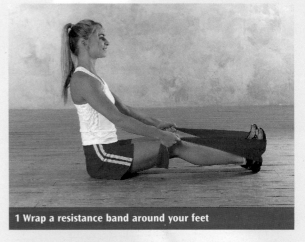

1 Wrap a resistance band around your feet

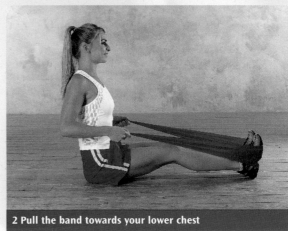

2 Pull the band towards your lower chest

11

Upright row

1 Stand with your feet one-and-a-half times hip-width apart, your bottom tucked under and your knees slightly bent. Hold your hand weights in front of you, with your palms facing your thighs and the ends of the weights almost touching.

2 Keeping the weights close to your body and leading the move with your elbows, raise the hand weights up to just below the level of your chin. Lower your arms under control back to the start position and repeat.

Do
Level one: one set of 12–16 reps
Level two: two sets of 12–16 reps

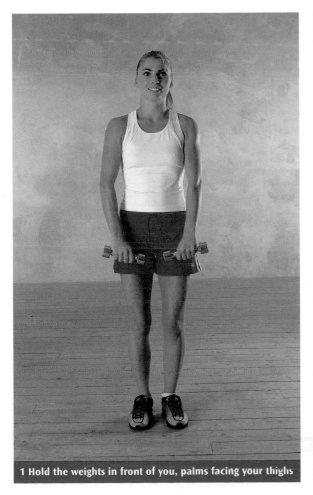

1 Hold the weights in front of you, palms facing your thighs

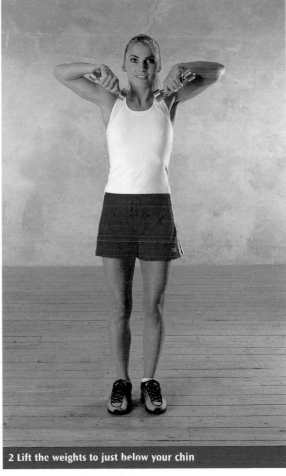

2 Lift the weights to just below your chin

Troubleshooting

Back extensions

1 Lie on your stomach with your hands flat on the floor, tucked in by your shoulders.

2 Slowly lift your head and upper body off the floor, supporting your weight with your hands. Keep your thighs and bottom relaxed (avoiding any tendency to tense up through the lower half of your body). Keep your abdominal muscles contracted as you lift. Slowly return to the floor and repeat.

Do

Level one: one set of 12–16 reps
Level two: two sets of 12–16 reps

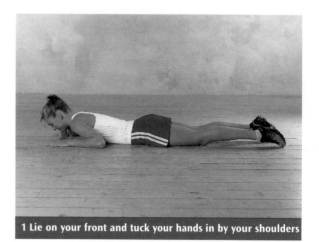

1 Lie on your front and tuck your hands in by your shoulders

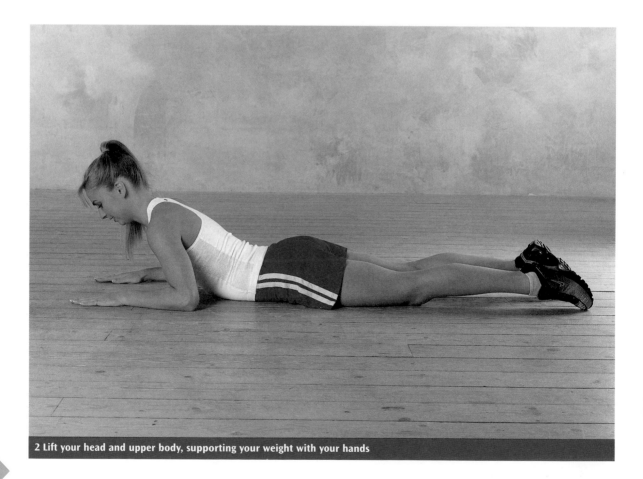

2 Lift your head and upper body, supporting your weight with your hands

11

One-arm row

1 Place your right hand and knee on a stable chair or bench. Extend your left foot to form a comfortable third point of a triangular base. This leg should be slightly bent. Take a hand weight in your left hand and extend (but don't lock) the arm downwards.

2 Keep your back straight, abdominals tight and look forward and slightly down. Draw your left arm up, leading the movement with the elbow and keeping the wrist straight. Bring the weight up towards your armpit, then lower under control. As you draw your arm up, think about squeezing your shoulder blades together and breathe out at the same time.

Do

Level one: one set of 12–16 reps
Level two: two sets of 12–16 reps

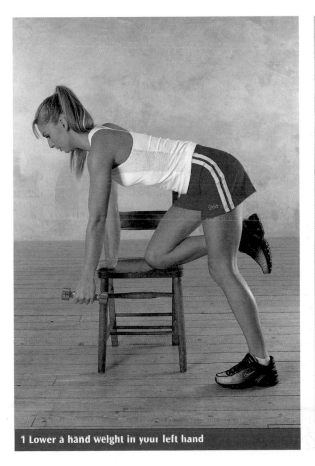

1 Lower a hand weight in your left hand

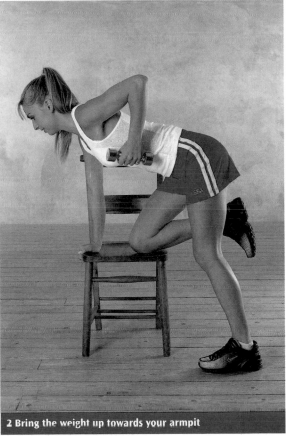

2 Bring the weight up towards your armpit

THE NEXT STEP

I hope this book has inspired you to delve further into the world of not just kick-boxing, but other martial arts too. There are many styles available; in fact it is usually the overwhelming proliferation of differing styles that puts people off. How can you even decide which one to study? Here is a brief overview and history of the most commonly available martial arts around.

Tai chi chuan

The initial aim of tai chi chuan is to teach the practitioner to relax. Not in the sense of lolling loosely around, but rather of using the body as efficiently as possible, with no muscular tension. Tai chi chuan incorporates chi kung exercises, which encourage deep breathing, improved blood circulation and a greater efficiency of all the body's systems. On a mental level, the calm concentration required for its practice can bring a serene state of mind – helpful in eradicating daily stresses and strains.

One of the most useful aspects of this martial art is that it is open to anyone. Age, health or infirmity are no barriers to practising tai chi and chi kung. However, to reach some of the higher levels does require some more demanding practice.

As a martial art, tai chi chuan works on a number of levels, but the principal aim is to teach practitioners to relax and become fluid in their movements. This helps them to acquire smoother actions and quicker response times. It is also occasionally referred to as internal kung fu. The 'internal' here refers to the general rule that tai chi chuan emphasizes the development of the internal aspects of the body – breathing, flexibility and the mind – as opposed to external tension or muscular strength.

The name itself is usually translated into English as 'the supreme ultimate fist'. The term 'tai chi' refers to the yin-yang symbol, which is highly prevalent in Chinese culture and more commonly known as the 'hard' and 'soft' sign – the two opposites coming together. The term 'chuan' refers to a boxing method – though in this context meaning a method of empty-hand combat, rather than a sporting contest. Therefore, as the name suggests, tai chi chuan is a self-defence method based on the Chinese Taoist philosophy of life.

The roots of tai chi chuan are shrouded in mystery and legend. It is said to have been created by the Taoist immortal Chang San-feng, a twelfth-century recluse who lived in the Wu-tang mountains, in the Hupeh Province of central China. He is said to have witnessed a fight between a snake and a crane, in which the crane's stabbing attack with its beak was neutralized by the snake's twisting elusive movements. He saw in this struggle living proof of the Taoist belief stated by the ancient master, Lao Tzu: 'The most yielding of things in the universe overcomes the most hard' (*Tao Te Ching*, verse 43).

Inspired by this, Chang San-feng created tai chi chuan. Charming as this story is, the roots of tai chi chuan are more likely to have been in Chen village, in the Honan Province. There are other styles of tai chi chuan, including the Yang style (founded by Yang Lu-chan, 1799–c. 1872), the Chen village style, the Sun style (founded by Sun Lu-t'ang, 1859–1933) and the Wu (founded by Wu Chien-chuan, 1870–1942). There is also a modern style of tai chi chuan developed on the mainland, which is gaining in popularity.

Tai chi chuan training includes punches, kicks, locks, open-hand techniques and throws in its repertoire, as well as the traditional Chinese weapons of the sword, broadsword, staff and spear. These days, the majority of people practise this art in order to improve and maintain their health and to provide a necessary antidote to the stresses and strains of modern life.

Tae kwon do

Tae kwon do (TKD) is derived from several martial arts, with the main influence being tae-kyon – Korean kick fighting. 'Tae' means 'kick' or 'smash with the feet'; 'kwon' means 'intercept' or 'strike with the hands'; and 'do' means 'the way of the art' – meaning that the foundation of the martial art is to use more than hands and feet to swiftly overcome your attacker.

TKD's origins stretch back over 2,000 years, and it is now practised by over 18 million people worldwide. It is an art of great range and contrast, and includes breathtaking leaping and flying kicks, originally evolved to enable a fighter on foot to unseat a warrior on horseback. During the 1950s, a group of leading martial-arts experts came together to unify what had previously been various disciplines into a single fighting system. This inauguration took place in South Korea on 11 April 1955, with Major-General Choi Hong Hi, a ninth Dan black belt, being credited as this newly unified martial arts founder. TKD spread worldwide from Korea in the 1960s, and the first World Tae Kwon Do Championship took place in Seoul, South Korea, in 1973. Since 1988, TKD has been listed as an Olympic sport.

At TKD clubs, trainees follow basic training on stance and guard, learning various movements, including blocks, punches, strikes and kicks. As training progresses, the patterns of stance become more diversified and complicated, allowing the simultaneous execution of two or more movements from the same position. This develops speed, power and flexibility, building into increasingly complicated patterns that allow a skilled exponent to attack enemies from every side.

TKD is quite a fast-moving martial art and is certainly a brilliant way to improve all-round fitness levels. However, if you have any joint, back or muscle injuries it would be wise to seek medical advice before taking part in any classes.

Karate

Karate, or karate-do, simply translated means 'empty hand' ('kara' means 'empty' and 'tc' means 'hand'), and this martial art is predominantly concerned with fighting with bare hands and feet. The basic principle is to turn the body into an effective weapon to defend and attack when and where appropriate.

Karate is now one of the most widely practised of the oriental martial arts. It evolved in the fifteenth century, during one of the Japanese occupations of the island of Okinawa, part of the Ryukyu chain of islands that runs between Japan and Taiwan. Its roots, however, can be traced much further back – all the way to ancient India. (Many people hold the view that the oriental martial arts have their roots in India. Indeed, when we look at disciplines such as yoga, there do seem to be great similarities.)

It is believed that Zen Buddhist monks took the Indian fighting techniques to China as early as the fifth and sixth centuries BC. Bodidharmi, the most famous of these monks, travelled at the end of the fifth century AD from India to China, where he became an instructor at the Shaolin monastery. He taught a combination of empty-hand fighting systems and yoga, and this became know as Shaolin Kung Fu – the system on which many Chinese martial arts systems are based.

In 1470, the Japanese had occupied the island of Okinawa. The law of the land dictated that anybody found carrying weapons would be put to death. In order to protect themselves from local bandits, who by and large ignored the prohibition on weapons, Zen Buddhist monks developed the empty-hand system known as te (hand). The new art was familiarly known as Okinawa-te (Okinawa hand). It was not until the twentieth century that it became known as karate-do.

Ju jitsu

The art of ju jitsu is interpreted as 'the science of softness'. Translated literally, 'ju' means 'soft' or 'gentle' and 'jitsu' means 'art'. Whilst referred to as a gentle art, some of the techniques taught are extremely dynamic and would appear to be anything but soft!

There are many stories regarding the origins of ju jitsu, dating back to the eighth century and earlier. While some people claim that ju jitsu originated in China, the ancient chronicles of Japan make reference to early 'empty hand' techniques. It is believed, however, that Ju Jitsu was bought to Japan by a Chinese monk called Chen Yuanein (1587–1671). So, although ju jitsu is viewed today as a Japanese martial art, there is strong evidence pointing to Chinese origins.

While ju jitsu was first practised in Japan by the samurai, followed by the ninja, it inevitably spread further afield and was, unfortunately, embraced by many of the bandits of the time. Through this dubious and unwanted association, ju jitsu earned a poor reputation. It was during this period that Jiguro Kano developed the art of judo (meaning 'the gentle way'), from a combination of ju jitsu techniques. His aim was to correct the reputation that ju jitsu had acquired.

The central philosophy behind ju jitsu is to conquer an opponent by all and any means - as long as minimal force is used. Another variation on ju jitsu that is gaining popularity is Brazilian ju jitsu. This emphasizes ground fighting – practitioners believe that since most fights end up on the ground, you might as well learn the most effective ground-fighting techniques available.

The introduction of ju jitsu to Brazil is largely credited to one Mitsuyo Maeda, who immigrated to Brazil in the 1920s and taught ju jitsu to Carlos Gracie of Rio de Janeiro. The large number of Japanese immigrants to South America ensured that traditional martial arts, including ju jitsu, would find a home in Latin America. However, Brazilian ju jitsu evolved into its own distinct style, honed in the rough *favelas* (shanty towns) of the big cities. No description of this form of ju jitsu is complete without mentioning the Gracie family. Carlos Gracie, after learning ju jitsu from Maeda, taught the art to his brothers Osvaldo, Gastao, Jorge and Helio. The Gracie family, through challenge matches, televised tournaments and sheer numbers, have spread their namesake style throughout the world.

Aikido

Created by Morihei Ueshiba (1883–1969), aikido in its present form is a relatively recent innovation within the martial-arts tradition. As a boy growing up in Japan, Ueshiba was introduced to the classical martial arts by his father, Yoroku. In 1912, Morihei moved to Hokkaido in northern Japan, where a chance meeting with a man called Sokaku Takeda changed his life.

Takeda was a master of daito ryu-aiki ju jitsu, a martial art that had originated in the sixth century AD and had been passed down throughout the military hierarchy and formalized by members of the Aizu clan, becoming known as oshikiuchi, or 'striking arts'. The young Ueshibi studied under Takeda until 1919. Then, on returning to his native Tanabe in the south on the death of his father, Morihei met Onisaburo Deguchi – the charismatic founder of an esoteric religion called omoto-kyo – and spent the next six years as his disciple, travelling throughout Asia.

In 1927, Morihei set up the Kobukan dojo in Tokyo and began teaching an amalgam of the martial traditions he had learned from Takeda, together with the spiritual beliefs he had gleaned from Deguchi. This new discipline, first known as Ueshiba aiko-budo, became aikido. This word is a combination of three concepts: 'ai' meaning 'harmony'; 'ki' meaning 'spirit'; and 'do' meaning 'way'. In a spiritual sense, this means harmonizing your individual spirit, or ki, with the spirit of nature itself. In the practical sense, this means that you harmonize with an attack, lead it to a point of exhaustion, and then neutralize it with a throw, a joint lock or an immobilization.

Aikido is a discipline that seeks not to meet violence with violence, but instead looks towards harmonizing with and restraining an opponent. Often recognized by the distinctive Hakama (a black skirt) which students are entitled to wear after passing their first Dan (black belt) exam, aikido training incorporates knife taking, sword and stick taking, and even defence from a kneeling position.

It is a martial art that can be learned for a variety of reasons: as a way of becoming physically fit, as self defence, or to understand something of Japanese culture. It is up to the individual to decide which area of the discipline to concentrate on.

Wing chun

Like aikido, wing chun kuen kung fu (commonly referred to as wing chun) can be considered a relative newcomer in the world of martial arts. The term 'wing chun' is attributed to a woman called Yin Wing Chun, who was a protégé of a Buddhist nun called Ng Mui. Wing chun is known as a soft style, but is in fact a blend of hard and soft techniques. A hard style involves meeting force with force, whereas a soft style employs more evasive manoeuvres and techniques.

Roughly translated, wing chun means 'beautiful springtime' and kuen means 'fist' or 'fist-fighting style'. Its blending of hard and soft styles is due to the fact that it was developed by a woman and refined mainly by men. It is centred on the Taoist principle of 'take the middle road'. In essence, this says that you should not go to extremes and that success is based on balance. If you are on the middle road you can see both the left and right paths, but if you venture too much to one side, you may lose sight of the other. This can also be interpreted as the concept yin and yang. Yin (the feminine side) focuses on diverting the flow of energy; yang (the masculine side) seeks to resist any opposing energy flow.

Wing chun, originally favoured by Bruce Lee before he created jeet kune do, features a characteristic turned-in style, with the body facing forwards. The hands protect the centre line and attack the opponent from close in. It is also well-known for its sticky-hands (chi sau) technique. To the uninitiated, this technique is best described as a hurt boxer trying to spoil his opponent's moves by clinging to his arms. The aim is to prevent an opponent striking freely, giving the wing-chun practitioner the opportunity to control, trap and break free to strike. The real skill lies in both parties wanting to achieve the same goal, and this has led to exceptional techniques, in which either one or both parties can train blindfolded.

Useful addresses

Umbrella organizations are good starting points for finding out what is available in your area.

UK

Amateur Martial Association
66 Chaddesden Lane
Chaddesden
Derby DE21 6LP
Tel: 01332 663086

British Council of Chinese Martial Arts
c/o 110 Frensham Drive
Stockingford
Nuneaton
Warwickshire CV10 9QL
Tel: 01203 394642

For information on my company and
its martial-arts teachers and personal
trainers, contact:
Fusion Fitness
annemarie36@btopenworld.com

For more information on personal
one-to-one training, contact:
Natasha Redfern
12 The Ridgedales
Coleridge Road
Oldham OL1 4RT
Tel: 07880 838 164

For more information on personal
one-to-one training and classes,
contact:
Master Martin Ace
The Martin Ace Black Belt Academy
77 Chichester Road
London N9 9DH
www.martinace.com
mail@martinace.com
Tel: 020 8345 5128

World Master Cris Janson Piers
cris@bfkko.co.uk or visit his website at
www.bfkko.co.uk
Tel: 07973 748907

Cris has his own successful
organizations in the BFKKO and the
WFKKO (world organization) and still
runs his own Falcon Martial Arts
Centres, but pays great respect to Mr
Tom Hibbert MBE of WAKO (World
Association of Kickboxing
Organizations) and AMA, who has
placed Cris as the National Full Contact
and Low Kick Coach to Great Britain.
Together they have produced many
champions and are proud of their
achievements.

Australia

Australian Martial Arts Association Inc.
PO Box 1272
McLaren Flat
SA 5171

Canada

For information on kick-boxing:
Jean Yves Theriault
c/o Instructors Dojo
259 Ste-Anne Street
Vanier
Ontario K1L 7C3
Tel: 613 746 5402

Jean Frenette
1075 Lionel Daunais
Boucherville
Quebec J4B 6V3
Tel: 450 449 7319

New Zealand

Try this website:
www.martial.co.nz

Index

Abdominal workout
  back extensions, 140
  heel touch, 140
  plank, the, 141
  sit up and twist, 141
  sit-ups, 139
Active lifestyle, 12
Aikido, 155
Arm workout
  bicep curl, 143
  hammer-head curls, 143
  lying triceps extensions, 142
  tricep kickbacks, 144

Bag gloves, 123
Basic metabolic rate, 11–13
Blood pressure, 37
Body fat
  excess, losing, 17
  lean body weight, balance of, 10
  meaning, 10
  measuring, 14
  monitors, 14
  range of, 14
Body image, 16
Body shapes, 15
Bottom workout
  bottom lift, 135
  glute raises, 135
  heel press, 133
  side kick, 134
Box-a-cise class, 86–91
Breakfast, 27, 28

Carbohydrates, 24
Cardiovascular fitness, 32–34
Cellulite, 13
Chest workout
  pec deck, 146
  press-ups, 147
  pull-overs, 147
  tricep dips, 145

Cholesterol levels, reducing, 37
Clothing, 47
Cross-trainers, 47
Crunches, 108
Cycling, 53

Dance, 54
Dieting see also Healthy Eating
  day-to-day eating, 26
  food diary, keeping, 21–23
  long-term weight loss, 18, 19
  losing weight, reasons for, 20
  weak points, 23
  yo-yo, 18
Drinking, 27

Ectomorph, 15
Endomorph, 15
Equipment, 48, 49, 123
Exercise see also Stretches
  blood pressure, reducing, 37
  cholesterol levels, reducing, 37
  cool-down, 44, 63–67
  feel-good factor, 37
  FITTA, 38
  glucose intolerance, reducing, 37
  illness, 40
  injury, 40
  maximum heart rate, 41, 42
  obesity, reducing, 37
  osteoporosis, prevention of, 37
  overload principle, 38
  pace, setting, 41, 42
  progression principle, 38
  pulse, taking, 42
  rate of perceived exertion, 41
  reasons for, 36
  relaxation and recuperation, 45

rest and recovery, 39
  specificity, 38, 39
  times for resting, 40
  training diary, 45
  warm-up, 43, 56–62
Exercise mat, 48

Fat, 24, 25
Fat-burn circuit class,
  crunches, 108
  press-ups, 106
  squat thrusts, 107
  star jumps, 110
  superman, 109
  workout, 104–111
Fighting stance, 69
Fish, 28
Fist, making, 68
Fitness
  aerobic, 34
  anaerobic, 34
  cardiovascular, 32–34
  flexibility, 32, 34, 35
  hip-to-waist ratio, 51
  level, assessing, 51
  meaning, 32
  motor, 32, 35
  muscular strength and endurance, 32, 34
  one-minute sit-up test, 51
  questionnaire, 50, 51
  step test, 51
Flexibility, 32, 34, 35
Focus mitts, 123
Food diary, 21
  conclusions, 23
  sample, 22
Fruit, 27

Glucose intolerance, 37

Hand weights, 48, 49
Hand wraps, 123
Healthy eating
  breakfast, 27, 28
  comfort eating, and, 31
  cravings, 31

day-to-day, 26
  eating out, 28
  eating when hungry, 30
  fish, 28
  fruit and vegetables, 27
  guidelines, 30
  lean, eating, 28, 29
  little and often, 28
  nutritional guidelines, 24, 25
  pigging out, and, 31
  portion control, 29
  seasonal, 27
  serving, meaning, 26
  snacks, 28
  water drinking, 27
Heart rate
  maximum, 41
  monitors, 42
Heavy back, 123
Heel digs, 59

Ju jitsu, 154, 155

Karate, 154
Kick-box class, 124–127
Kick-boxing
  basics, 68–73
  clothing, 47
  equipment, 48, 49, 123
  hybrid sport, as, 7
  modern system of, 8
  place for, 46
  stance, 69
Kicking
  safe, 71, 72
  targets, 72, 76
Kicking shields, 123
Kicks and punches
  aerobic kicks, 96, 98, 102, 114
  axe kick-round kick-jab-cross, 116
  axe kicks, 96
  cross, 76
  front and rear elbow, 85
  front kick, 79

front kick-jab-cross, 83
front kick-round kick, 100
front-leg round kick, 99
hook, 78
hook-hook-roundhouse, 130
jab, 76
jab-cross, 77
jab-cross-front kick, 128
jab-cross-hook-uppercut, 93
jab-cross-rear knee strike, 97
jab-cross-rear knee strike-
  round kick, 119
jab-overhand-body hook,
  121
jab-roundhouse, 82
jab-spinning back fist, 94
jab-spinning back fist-cross,
  120
jumping front kicks, 114,
  118
left hook-right hook, 88
left hook-right uppercut, 89
left jab-left uppercut, 90
left jab-right cross, 87
left uppercut-right uppercut,
  88
low roundhouse-high
  roundkick, 95
overhand, 121
right hook-left uppercut, 90
right jab-right uppercut, 91
round kick-jab-cross-rear-leg
  front kick, 112
roundhouse kick, 80
side kicks, 81, 98
side knees, 102
uppercut, 84
Knee bends, 59
Knee lifts, 58
Kung fu, 8
Kyikushinkai karate, 8
Kyokky shinkai, 8

Lateral raises, 129
Leg curls, 60
Lunges, 131, 136

Marching, 58
Martial arts, popularity of, 8
Mesomorph, 15
Motor fitness, 32, 35
Muay Thai, 7–9
Muscle, weight of, 13

Neck rolls, 59

Obesity, reducing, 37
Osteoporosis, 37

Pad and bag work, 122, 123
Pec deck, 131
Pelvic circles, 60
Physiotherapy, 50
Pivoting, 73
Plank, the, 141
Pregnancy, 40
Press-ups, 106, 147
Protein, 25
Pulse, taking, 42
Punching, 70

Racket sports, 53
Resistance bands, 49
Running, 52, 53

Salt, 25
Sedentary lifestyle, 12
Shin pads, 123
Shoulder rolls, 58
Side steps, 60
Sit-ups, 139
Skin-fold callipers, 14
Skipping rope, 48
Sparring gloves, 123
Squat thrusts, 107
Squats, 129
Star jumps, 110
Stretches, 44
  back and side, 61, 67
  benefits of, 57
  calf, 62, 64
  chest and front-shoulders,
    61
  cool-down, 64–67

glute, 65
hamstring, 62
hip-flexor, 65
inner thigh, 66
lower-back ball, 65
lying quad, 64
quad, 62
quick routine, 67
re-energizing jumps, 67
seated chest, 66
seated hamstring, 64
shoulder, 67
tower, 66
trapezius, 61
tricep, 66
warm up, 57
Superman, 109
Sweating, 39
Swimming, 53

Tae kwon-do, 6–8, 104, 153
Tai chi chuan, 152, 153
Thai boxing, 7–9
Thai pads, 123
Thigh workout
  hip opener, 138
  inside thigh, 138
  lunges, 136
  straight leg lifts, 137
Troubleshooting, 132–151

Upper-back workout
  back extensions, 150
  one arm row, 151
  seated row, 148
  upright row, 149

Vegetables, 27

Walking, 52
Warm-up, 43
  heel digs, 59
  knee bends, 59
  knee lifts, 58
  leg curls, 60
  marching, 58
  neck rolls, 59

pelvic circles, 60
shoulder rolls, 58
side steps, 60
stretching, 57, 61, 62
Water, drinking, 27
Weight control, 6
Weight loss
  eating habits, changing, 30
  goal-setting, 30
  motivation, 20
  reasons for, 20
Weight versus size, 13
Wing chun, 156
Workouts see also Stretches
  abdominal, 139–141
  advanced, 112–121
  arm, 142–144
  beginners', 76–85
  bottom, for, 133–135
  box-a cise class, 86–91
  cardio breaks, 43
  chest, 145–147
  combined, building, 55
  cool-down, 44, 63–67
  cross-training, 52–55
  fat-burn circuit class,
    104–111
  grace, acquiring, 74
  intermediate, 92–103
  kick-boxing and cardio
    breaks, 43
  levels, 74
  quick, 128–131
  thigh, 136–139
  timing, 75
  training diary, 45
  troubleshooting, 44
  upper-back, 148–151
  warm-up, 43, 56–62

Author's acknowledgements

Cassie White

Although it was her first time modelling, she took to it like a professional – thank you for your time and effort and for helping make the kick-boxing workouts look so perfect.

Natasha Redfern

Thank you for your many visits to London and your good humour in always having to get up at the crack of dawn to get to our photo shoots. Your help was much appreciated.

Kerry-Louise Norbury and Master Cris Janson Piers

Again thank you for all your time, effort and advice in the making of this book. It was a pleasure working with you both.

Master Martin Ace

My friend and teacher was his usual patient and helpful self, giving me his time and expertise without question. Thank you.

Tabitha

A thank you to my daughter Tabitha, who though like her mother insisted on being early, still had the decency to wait to the day after I finished writing this book!

Finally to my mother-in-law Gillian Jacob, my sister-in-law Dawn White and my mother. Thank you for all the help you have both given me during my pregnancy and in Tabitha's first few months – without which I would never had had enough time or sleep to complete any work whatsoever.

The publishers would also like to thank Casalls (c/o Viva (UK) Limited, 2 Market Place, Somerton, Somerset, TA11 7LX) for kindly lending sports clothes for the photoshoots, and Tao Sports, 523 Green Lanes, London N4 for the loan of kick-boxing equipment. All photography by Donna Eaves except pages 7, 8 and 9 by Tim Winter, pages 11, 12, 17, 47, 50 , 52, 53, 54 and 132 courtesy of PhotoDisc and pages 35, 36–7, 39 and 44 courtesy of ImageState.